Advances in Cancer Nanotheranostics for Experimental and Personalized Medicine

Edited by

Prof. Dr. Yusuf TUTAR

University of Health Sciences,
Hamidiye Health Sciences Institute,
Division of Molecular Medicine
34668, Istanbul,
Turkey

and

Department of Basic Pharmaceutical Sciences,
University of Health Sciences,
Hamidiye Faculty of Pharmacy,
Division of Biochemistry
34668, Istanbul,
Turkey

Advances in Cancer Nanotheranostics for Experimental and Personalized Medicine

Editor: Yusuf Tutar

ISBN (Online): 978-981-14-5691-6

ISBN (Print): 978-981-14-5689-3

ISBN (Paper Back): 978-981-14-5690-9

© 2020, Bentham Books imprint.

Published by Bentham Science Publishers Pte. Ltd. Singapore. All Rights Reserved.

need for a court order if at any point you breach any terms of this License Agreement. In no event will any delay or failure by Bentham Science Publishers in enforcing your compliance with this License Agreement constitute a waiver of any of its rights.

3. You acknowledge that you have read this License Agreement, and agree to be bound by its terms and conditions. To the extent that any other terms and conditions presented on any website of Bentham Science Publishers conflict with, or are inconsistent with, the terms and conditions set out in this License Agreement, you acknowledge that the terms and conditions set out in this License Agreement shall prevail.

Bentham Science Publishers Pte. Ltd.
80 Robinson Road #02-00
Singapore 068898
Singapore
Email: subscriptions@benthamscience.net

BENTHAM SCIENCE

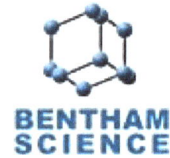

CONTENTS

FOREWORD

Oncologic drug development focused on single target-single drug strategy for several years. However, cancer cells are genius! They can bypass inhibitor perturbations by using alternative routes. Further, human genome project results indicated that four letter-alphabet is not as simple as central dogma; only few percent of the gene sequences are transcribed and translated. Rest of the genome function is involved in uncharacterized biochemical pathways and cell biology. And epigenetics and metabolites add more complexity to the understanding of molecular mechanisms in detail. This unknown mechanism makes cancer cell genius!!! But a great endeavor of eminent scientists and continuous research to elucidate pathways both in cellular and tissue levels make drug design more effective every day.

To control the effect of several cellular factors, the new trend in contemporary drug design is to employ drug cocktail that will synergistically act on these factors and proper oncologic drug targeting to eliminate off-targeting. For this purpose, nanocarriers have been designed to deliver drugs to tumor microenvironment not only to treat the tumor but prevent its metastasis.

Biomimicking is an old fashioned yet excellent method in disease treatment. Macrophages target cancer cells and using this biomimick bullet macromolecule with oncologic drug cargo serves as a fine treatment strategy. The biomimick bullet cargo can be a wide range of molecules from small to large molecules.

Targeting with nanotheranostic carriers provides specific delivery to cancer microenvironment. However, cancer cells so called "the other strategies" yet to be elucidated. For example, transformation of a healthy cell to cancer cell may enhance inner and surface signaling molecules and may introduce new set of metabolites. Further, some of the non-coding gene's expression increases during this transformation. Altogether, cellular and tissue level characterization of oncologic pathways may help our understanding of tumor biology. Currently, cancer nanotheranostics tries to find a short cut for experimental and personalized medicine in cancer treatment. This book covers recent advances in this field.

Prof Lütfi TUTAR
Ahi Evran University
Turkey

PREFACE

Personalized medicine with novel therapeutic approaches provides direct targeting of macromolecules with contemporary drug delivery systems for treatment of severe diseases, including cancer. Nanotheranostic design offers increased bioavailability of the drugs through controlled release and distribution. Nanotheranostics also integrates diagnostic test with treatment of the disease. Recent advances in cancer studies revealed new genetic elements and factors that affect theranostic drug targeting approaches. Also, several tumors are challenging, and new treatment modalities are required. Molecular level mechanisms provide valuable information for therapy and innovative design for treatment. Several creative approaches have been proposed for theranostic therapy. For this reason, an updated approach over *in vivo* and translational properties of nanotheranostics with special emphasis on cancer will widen the scope of the readers/researchers with this book.

Chapter 1 despite significant advances in cancer therapy, many tumors are still challenging, and novel strategies are essential for treatment. Nanotheranostics use nanotechnology for diagnosis and therapy of cancer. Recent advancement in nanotechnology has provided novel types of nanomaterials composed of either organic- or polymer-based nanoparticles. Small alterations and modifications transform this carrier system with unique properties and optimize drug delivery and release. This chapter provides overview in cancer nanotheranostics field.

Chapter 2 overviews tumor microenvironment as prelude. This site regulates tumor progression and metastasis. Non-cellular components in this environment such as cytokines, chemokines, growth factors, inflammatory and matrix remodeling enzymes shape the progression of the disease by mediating the communication taking place between the tumor itself and its surrounding. This may prevent the benefits of therapeutical strategies. The chapter focuses on understanding the function and mechanism of these non-cellular components in the environment to elucidate obstacles in the treatment of cancer.

Chapter 3 covers immune system employment in fighting cancer cells to prevent tumor development. Immunotherapies are innovative cancer treatment. Nanomedical formulations modulate macrophages which can influence the tumor microenvironment, since macrophages target tumor environment. Macrophage may be used as trojan horse and its cargo may mediate gene and/or protein expression in the treatment regime. This section discusses improvements in cancer immunotherapies through this biological strategy.

Chapter 4 Gene and genome modification tools allow gene therapy through alteration of malignant genes and editing mutations for correction of errors. These innovative technologies deliver therapeutic nucleic acids to cells and tissues. Therefore, the success of gene therapy formulation is proportional to efficient delivery of the carrier and its nucleic acid cargo to a specific target and proper cellular uptake. The platforms have been developed for higher loading capacity, and low immunogenicity and toxicity. In chapter 4, the authors provide a review on different gene delivery vectors and platforms at the nanoscale.

Chapter 5 Oncology research applications may not yet fully suppress cancer-based mortalities and morbidities. Conventional therapeutic approaches have limitations as most research depends on coding genes. Human genome sequencing revealed that only 2-3 percent of the genome codes for genes and proteins however the rest is unknown. Further, heterogeneity among malignant tumors lead obstacles. Therefore, "precision medicine" in oncology and its extrapolation to "personalized treatment" for each cancer patient is essential. The chapter covers non-coding RNAs as biopharmaceutical tools in oncology. The new trend in drug design is covered in this section.

Chapter 6 Nanoparticles are convenient carrier systems based on their plasmonic and magnetic properties, active surface areas and various physicochemical properties. Development of therapeutic nanoparticles provides imaging modalities such as magnetic resonance imaging, radionuclide-based imaging; positron emission tomography and single-photon emission computed tomography and X-ray-computed tomography. Methodology and applications of the techniques are explained thoroughly in this chapter.

Chapter 7 covers practical clinical applications in chemotherapy and nuclear medicine. The simultaneous yield of imaging in radiologic and nuclear medicine applications and therapeutic agents offers diagnosis and treatment effectiveness in real-time.

This book covers recent advancements both in applied and in clinical research. Since targeting small organic molecules are common, the book mainly focused on DNA, protein and immunotherapy on cancer. Different applications for cancer treatment are in progress but basic strategies are similar. We hope this book will help not only early career scientists but also will help experienced researchers to widen the scope of their projects.

Yusuf TUTAR
University of Health Sciences
Istanbul
Turkey

List of Contributors

Ezgi Nurdan Yenilmez Tunoglu	University of Health Sciences, Hamidiye Health Sciences Institute, Division of Molecular Medicine, 34668, Istanbul, Turkey
Berçem Yeman	University of Health Sciences, Hamidiye Health Sciences Institute, Division of Molecular Medicine, 34668, Istanbul, Turkey
Merve Biçen	University of Health Sciences, Hamidiye Health Sciences Institute, Division of Molecular Medicine, 34668, Istanbul, Turkey
Servet Tunoglu	Department of Molecular Medicine, Aziz Sancar Institute of Experimental Medicine, Istanbul University, 34093, Istanbul, Turkey
Yousef Rasmı	Department of Biochemistry, Faculty of Medicine, Urmia University of Medical Sciences, 571478334, Urmia, Iran
Yusuf Tutar	University of Health Sciences, Hamidiye Health Sciences Institute, Division of Molecular Medicine, 34668, Istanbul, Turkey University of Health Sciences, Hamidiye Faculty of Pharmacy, Department of Basic Pharmaceutical Sciences, Division of Biochemistry, 34668, Istanbul, Turkey
Raghda Ashraf Soliman	Pharmaceutical Biology Department, Faculty of Pharmacy and Biotechnology, German University in Cairo, 11835, Cairo, Egypt
Rana Ahmed Youness	Pharmaceutical Biology Department, Faculty of Pharmacy and Biotechnology, German University in Cairo, 11835, Cairo, Egypt
Mohamed Zakaria Gad	Biochemistry Department, Faculty of Pharmacy and Biotechnology, German University in Cairo, 11835, Cairo, Egypt
Asmaa Mostafa	Department of Internal Medicine III, University Hospital RWTH Aachen, Pauwelsstraße 30, 52074, Aachen, Germany Department of Microbial Biotechnology, Division of Genetic Engineering and Biotechnology, National Research Center, 33 El-Bohouth St., El-Dokki, 12622, Giza, Egypt
Matthias Bartneck	Department of Internal Medicine III, University Hospital RWTH Aachen, Pauwelsstraße 30, 52074, Aachen, Germany
Beatriz B. Oliveira	UCIBIO, Life Sciences Department, Faculdade de Ciências e Tecnologia, Campus de Caparica, 2829-516 Caparica, Portugal
Alexandra R. Fernandes	UCIBIO, Life Sciences Department, Faculdade de Ciências e Tecnologia, Campus de Caparica, 2829-516 Caparica, Portugal
Pedro V. Baptista	UCIBIO, Life Sciences Department, Faculdade de Ciências e Tecnologia, Campus de Caparica, 2829-516 Caparica, Portugal
Seda Keleştemur	University of Health Sciences, Institution of Health Sciences, Department of Biotechnology, Tıbbiye Cad., 34668, Istanbul, Turkey
Gamze Kuku	Yeditepe University, Faculty of Engineering, Department of Genetics and Bioengineering, Kayısdagı Cad., 34755, Istanbul, Turkey
Turkan Ikizceli	Department of Radiology, University of Health Sciences Turkey, Haseki Training and Research Hospital, Istanbul, Turkey

S. Karacavus   Department of Nuclear Medicine, University of Health Sciences Turkey, Kayseri City Training and Research Hospital, Kayseri, Turkey

CHAPTER 1

Cancer Nanotheranostics

Ezgi Nurdan Yenilmez Tunoglu[1], Berçem Yeman[1], Merve Biçen[1], Servet Tunoglu[2], Yousef Rasmi[3] and Yusuf Tutar[1,4,*]

[1] *University of Health Sciences, Hamidiye Health Sciences Institute, Division of Molecular Medicine, 34668, Istanbul, Turkey*

[2] *Department of Molecular Medicine, Aziz Sancar Institute of Experimental Medicine, Istanbul University, 34093, Istanbul, Turkey*

[3] *Department of Biochemistry, Faculty of Medicine, Urmia University of Medical Sciences, 571478334, Urmia, Iran*

[4] *Department of Basic Pharmaceutical Sciences, University of Health Sciences, Hamidiye Faculty of Pharmacy, Division of Biochemistry, 34668, Istanbul, Turkey*

Abstract: Molecular profiling of diseases identifies specific cancer-causing genes and associated networks. Administered drug displays different therapeutic efficiency depending on individual cancer subtype and therapeutic responses. Personalized medicine helps designing treatment methods for individual patients with distinct diseases. For complete understanding of patient's pathophysiology, different omics data types are integrated. These data can be derived from whole-exome sequencing, metabolomics, pharmacogenomics, and proteomics. Pharmacogenomics deals with the interaction of drug and patient's genetic make-up and metabolomics reveals custom regulation of biochemical pathways in patients. Transcriptomics and proteomics analyze organism tissue or cell type in cancer and play even more relevant role in personalized medicine. Since associated genetic anomalities and metabolic profiles influence therapy response, a continuous evolution of cancer nanotheranostics helps preventing and treating the disease more precisely.

Keywords: Cancer, Metabolomics, Nanotheranostics, Personalized medicine.

INTRODUCTION

There is a six million nucleotide difference between two individual's genome and even twins have 35 intergenerational mutational nucleotide differences [1]. Epigenetic alterations as well as gene duplication or deletion like unequal crossing over alter genomic content during the course of individual life cycle.

---

[*] **Corresponding author Yusuf Tutar:** University of Health Sciences, Hamidiye Health Sciences Institute, Division of Molecular Medicine, 34668, Istanbul, Turkey and Department of Basic Pharmaceutical Sciences, University of Health Sciences, Hamidiye Faculty of Pharmacy, Division of Biochemistry, 34668, Istanbul, Turkey;
E-mail: yusuf.tutar@sbu.edu.tr

Therefore, nanotheranostic approaches require delivery of individually adapted medicine based on genetic profiles of cancer patients. High-throughput technologies in oncology provide genomic analysis to be used for guidance of individualized medical treatment.

Initial studies of individualized treatment started with the Human Genome Project (HGP). HGP has helped to make use of the relationship between drug and target and improve its efficacy and safety. In this concept, patients are individually treated taking their unique genomic profiles into consideration. Even though the genomic profiles of different cells of a patient are the same, their expression profiles are clearly different. This difference is taken into account in personalized medicine along with the patient's disease history. On the other hand, traditional treatment methods have overlooked the genetic variability among patients and focused on a reactive approach based on population-based conclusions. During the physical examination; symptoms described by patients, medications taken, and biopsy outcomes are taken into account to decide on the traditional method to be implemented [2].

A new concept, P4 medicine, was first introduced in 2011 by Hood *et al.* as a systems approach including predictive, preventive, personalized, and participatory features of medicine. This approach puts emphasis on the patient instead of the disease itself, making it a proactive discipline rather than reactive [3]. P4 medicine does not focus just on genomic data but also involves data from DNA (together with epigenetic changes), RNA, protein, metabolite, cell, and tissue level. Using the data gathered, it is possible to personalize any form of treatment for any form of disease. It is important to have as much knowledge as possible of each patient's and tumor's genetic backgrounds to increase the efficiency of targeted treatment. When the two pieces of information are evaluated with regard to one another, it is also possible to determine the risk groups for specific disease types. Overall, personalized medicine aims to design the right treatment for the right patient at the right time and the right dose.

Oncology in Brief

Our body is a living and growing system that contains billions of cells that perform many functions such as metabolism, transport, secretion, reproduction and mobility. Growth and development occur as a result of the growth of newly formed cells and their transformation into different types of tissues. The branch of oncology is interested in cancer and the biochemistry of cancer cells is different. There are three different types of cells in our body: static cells (differentiated cells), growing cells (undifferentiated cells) and regenerating cells (stem cells). In contrast to these cell types, cancer cells do not have a growth-inhibiting control mechanism as in normal cells. Therefore, it is possible to compare cancer cells to uncontrolled stem cells. Tumors can be malignant or benign tumors. Cancer occurs due to many factors. In addition to genetic factors, many environmental factors such as UV light, X-rays, chemicals and tobacco products can cause cancer. In order to define cancer, it is necessary to understand cancer genetics. There are three types of genes in cancer genetics: Oncogenes, tumor suppressors and DNA repair genes. The normal form of an oncogene is defined as a proto-oncogene. Proto-oncogenes are converted to oncogenes by mutation. Tumor suppressors produce proteins that avoid cell division and cause cell death. Genes that prevent cancer-causing mutations are DNA repair genes. Occasionally, a virus-induced mechanism inserts nucleotides into or near a proto-oncogene and transform it to an oncogene. This results in uncontrolled cell growth. A single oncogene is usually not adequate to cause cancer. Cancer-related genes [4] serve as a biomarker in the definition of cancer (Table **1**).

Table 1. Some genes associated with cancer.

Name	Function	Examples of Cancer/Diseases	Type of Cancer Gene
APC	regulates transcription of target genes	Familial Adenomatous Polyposis	tumor suppressor
BCL2	involved in apoptosis; stimulates angiogenesis	Leukemia; Lymphoma	oncogene
BLM	DNA repair	Bloom Syndrome	DNA repair
BRCA1	may be involved in cell cycle control	Breast, Ovarian, Prostatic, & Colonic Neoplasms	tumor suppressor
BRCA2	DNA repair	Breast & Pancreatic Neoplasms; Leukemia	tumor suppressor
HER2	tyrosine kinase; growth factor receptor	Breast, Ovarian Neoplasms	oncogene
MYC	involved in protein-protein interactions with various cellular factors	Burkitt's Lymphoma	oncogene
p16	cyclin-dependent kinase inhibitor	Leukemia; Melanoma; Multiple Myeloma; Pancreatic Neoplasms	tumor suppressor
p21	cyclin-dependent kinase inhibitor		tumor suppressor
p53	apoptosis; transcription factor	Colorectal Neoplasms; Li-Fraumeni Syndrome	tumor suppressor

(Table 1) cont.....

Name	Function	Examples of Cancer/Diseases	Type of Cancer Gene
RAS	GTP-binding protein; important in signal transduction cascade	Pancreatic, Colorectal, Bladder Breast, Kidney, & Lung Neoplasms; Leukemia; Melanoma	oncogene
RB	regulation of cell cycle	Retinoblastoma	tumor suppressor
SIS	growth factor	Dermatofibrosarcoma; Meningioma; Skin Neoplasms	oncogene
XP	DNA repair	Xeroderma pigmentosum	DNA repair

Another term in cancer biology is "angiogenesis". Angiogenesis is the process by which new capillary blood vessels are formed to supplement blood cells with nutrients and oxygen. Without angiogenesis, tumors cannot exceed half the size of one mm. In the treatment of cancer, surgical intervention, radiotherapy, chemotherapy, and immunotherapy methods are used.

The cancer pathway is a system of regulation in which activation or inactivation by a genetic or epigenetic mutation is required for the development of cancer. Janus Kinases (JAKS), the JAKS/STAT pathway generated by signal transducers and transcription activators (STATs), play an important role in mediating cell fate such as apoptosis, differentiation and proliferation in response to growth factor and cytokines. Disruption of the JAK/STAT signaling pathway contributes to tumorigenesis. STAT3 is active in more than 50% of lung and breast cancer tumors; in over 95% of head and neck cancers. The JAK/STAT signaling pathway also regulates the cellular response to cytokines and attenuated STAT signaling. The notch signaling pathway plays an important role in tissue homeostasis. The notch can inhibit the spread of cellular differentiation within a tissue. T-cell acute leukemia is a type of blood cancer that results from the unlimited proliferation of immature T-cells. Abnormal Notch signal is not only observed in this type of cancer, but also in breast cancer, ovarian cancer and brain tumors. It is possible that the signals in the Notch signaling pathway may enhance cell proliferation by downstream activation of the transcription factor C-myc, where impaired expressions are observed in many cancer types. The RAS-Mitogen-activated Protein Kinase (MAPK) signaling pathway constitutes an important part of the translation of signals from cytokines and growth factors. Mutations in this signaling pathway occurred in approximately 45% of colon cancer and approximately 90% of pancreatic cancer. Similar to the MAPK signaling pathway, the phosphatidylinositol 3-kinase/AKT (PI3K/AKT) signaling pathway responds to various extra and intracellular signals transmitted by hormonal receptors, tyrosine-kinase-bound receptors, and intracellular factors. The PI3K/AKT signaling pathway is active in many types of cancer. Activation of this signaling pathway promotes cell survival and proliferation. The nuclear factor kappa B (NF-kB) signaling pathway regulates genes involved in key cellular processes such as proliferation, stress response, hereditary immunity, and inflammation. Signals in this signaling pathway are activated by many extracellular factors such as tumor necrosis factor, interleukin, growth factors, bacterial and viral infections, oxidative stress, and pharmaceutical compounds. Disruption of this pathway results in malignant tumors in human B cells. The Wnt signaling pathway consists of calcium, planar polarity and standard portion. Distortion in the standard part results in colon cancer and breast cancer. Homeostatic displacement occurs in many epithelia of the human body. The Wnt signaling path plays an important role in this process. Abnormal Wnt signaling results in chronic and acute myeloid leukemia. The TGF-β signaling pathway was first discovered in tumors as an anti-proliferation signal that controls tissue proliferation and provides tissue homeostasis. Similar to the Wnt signal path, this path includes SMAD1/5/8, SMAD2/3, and TAB/TAK. Activation of this signaling pathway takes place with TGF-β ligands that bind to the extracellular portion of TGF-β receptors. Mutations, reduced regulation of TGF-β receptors, inactivation of SMAD4 are found in many types of cancer. Inactivation of SMAD4 results in approximately 53% pancreatic adenocarcinomas [5].

CD36 (platelet integral membrane glycoprotein IV) is known as a suitable receptor for thrombospondin-1 (TSP-1). TSP-1 protease activity in extracellular matrices and platelet granules is involved in TGF-β activation, regulation of neurite outgrowth and angiogenesis, as well as cell addition, mobility, proliferation. Lipid metabolism has attracted interest from researchers in this area in terms of tumor onset, development and important role in metastasis. CD36 can be used as an important cancer-targeted biomarker in lipid homeostasis, angiogenesis, immune response, adhesion, and metastasis in cancer. CD36 plays an important role in regulating endothelial cell function in multiple cancer types, such as brain tumor, colorectal and breast cancer. High density lipoprotein (HDL) is known to have anticancer effects, while low density lipoprotein (LDL) cannot be ruled out. CD36 has been reflected in studies where it acts as a scavenger regarding LDL. The deterioration of lipid metabolism and inflammation causes oxidative stress to produce oxidized LDL (oxLDL). A high-fat diet can cause cancer. OxLDL levels were higher in patients with cancer (breast, ovarian) than non-cancer patients. CD36 and LOX-1 (lectin-like receptor) are important in the uptake of oxLDL. Cholesterol homeostasis is maintained in part by cells that express the radical scavenging receptors (CD36) then absorb oxLDL, which are then converted to oxysterol ligands of nuclear liver X receptors. Heterodimers of activated liver X receptors (LXR) target genes with the LXR element containing ATP binding transporters leading to cholesterol efflux to HDL or cholesterol release by the intestines. While oxLDL can reduce chemodynamic sensitivity to drugs such as cisplatin, statin therapy can lower serum oxLDL. Also, statins are important in the regulation of radical scavenging receptors in oxidative pathways [6 - 11].

Autophagy is a catabolic process that is maintained by the vesicle and maintains homeostatic functions such as protein degradation and organelle turnover, which is degraded in the lysosome. This mechanism eliminates hazardous compounds such as cytostatic compounds and harmful organelles [6 - 11]. A disorder in autophagy will cause tumor growth. Many autophagy-related inhibitors can be used to inhibit the growth of tumors [12]. However, tumor heterogeneity, quantitative degree of autophagy, and duration of drug administration are the points to be considered in this case.

A high enough *de novo* biosynthesis rate in cancer may not always be possible; for example, in solid tumors, enlargement and inadequate vascularization may limit glucose and oxygen delivery. If oxygen is limited, the activation of the hypoxia inducible factor 1 (HIF1) pathway may increase survival [6 - 11].

Effective cancer treatment is still a major challenge for modern medicine. Nanotechnology has tremendous potential to improve cancer treatment. Lipid-based formulations, poly (ethylene glycol) (PEG), polyamidoamine (PAMAM), dextran-based platforms, gold NPs, quantum dots can be used as drug delivery systems [13]. Multidrug resistance is an important concern in cancer [14]. There are studies where siRNA and anticancer drugs are given to cancer cells simultaneously. While siRNA silences the relevant genes involved in drug resistance, accumulation of anticancer drug in cancer cells gives chemotherapeutic results following the release of siRNA.

Genomic Era

Human Genome Project (HGP) put a new dimension to patient therapy, disease diagnostic, and drug design research. Advances in technology, from past to present, have allowed the analysis of complex biological systems and, accurate identification of early diagnostic factors of diseases. Sequencing technologies have helped to interpret the genetic code of various organisms. The knowledge gained after the completion of HGP has altered the perspective of genomics. Genomic approaches focus on the diagnosis of diseases in order to predict the risk of patients for various diseases. Cancer-specific mutations can be an example of genomic approaches in the clinic. As an example, in patients with non-polyposis colorectal cancer, Lynch Syndrome is caused by mutations in DNA mismatch repair genes like MLH1, PMS1 [15]. Mutations in BRCA1 and BRCA2 genes often cause hereditary ovary and breast cancer [16]. Even though different individuals may have the same tumor type, they may have different mutations such as single nucleotide polymorphism (SNP), deletion/insertion and copy number variations. All these differences have led researchers to identify early indicators of cancer. In the light of new technologies, genetic mapping plays a critical role of deciding on treatment options that vary among patients. Next Generation Sequencing (NGS) allows sequencing individual tumor DNA, including single-cell level sequencing as well. Analyzing the data set generated from sequencing points out the number and profile of somatic mutations in a patient that can be different. Therefore, personalized medicine catches growing attention, and has become nearly necessary for individual treatment planning. Genomic technologies in pharmacology are used to predict individual responses to any given drug. Until today, many pharmacogenomic tests have been developed for clinical use. For example, maintenance of oral anticoagulant warfarin dose is associated with 2 genes, CYP2C9 and VKORC1 [17]. Consideration of the CYP2C9 genotype together with VKORC1 helps determine the necessary warfarin dose. Despite the accumulated genomic information, many obstacles must be handled to use this information in medicinal applications.

Transcriptome Analysis

Since DNA sequencing and microarray technologies advanced, profiling and analyzing the transcriptome have become a useful tool to determine molecular mechanisms underlying cancer development and progression. Growing transcriptome dataset has allowed us to associate between DNA sequence variations and gene expression changes. Until today, Gene Expression Omnibus (GEO) database has collected approximately 800K sets of transcriptomic data. Numerous researches have shown the gene expression pattern that can guide clinicians to predict treatment responses. As a result of these datasets, many clinical tests have improved the prediction of prognosis and relapse risk for patients with a variety of cancers, such as breast, colorectal, and non-small lung cancer [18 - 20].

Recently, extended studies at the single-cell level have helped increase our knowledge of cell or tumor complexity in cancer and this may influence clinicians to decide on treatment options in terms of personalized medicine.

Epigenomic Regulations

Even though differences in somatic mutations, germline factors, and gene expression profiles help us understand the characterization of cancer cells or tumors, in recent years, researchers have focused on how gene expressions are regulated in tissues and cells. This regulation mechanism called epigenetics plays an important role in tumor formation and growth. Epigenetic regulations clarify the alterations in DNA methylation, histone modification, and non-coding RNA function (miRNAs, lnRNAs) [21 - 23]. These differences are thought to affect cancer drug response. Some research is ongoing for epigenetic mechanisms in cancer. For example, methylation status of MGMT promotor is evaluated to see whether temozolamide (a DNA alkylating agent) will be an efficient drug for treatment of glioblastoma [24]. Elevated levels of miRNA-449a have been revealed to increase the survival rate in chemotherapy-treated triple-negative breast cancer patients [25]. As a histone deacetylase 8 inhibitor, PCI-34051 induced apoptosis in a calcium-mediated manner and has shown promising results in preclinical studies for treating T-cell malignancies [26]. In conclusion, all these epigenetic alterations may help understand the drug resistance mechanisms in patients undergoing chemotherapy.

Proteomic Approaches

Although genomics and transcriptomics are very useful tools, they are not enough to clarify the mechanisms underlying human diseases. Therefore, we need to do further studies to explore cellular mechanisms. Central dogma of molecular biology explains clearly that RNAs are transcribed from DNA, proteins are translated from RNA. Proteins, the translational products of RNA, are the main components of cellular functions. Posttranslational modifications and conformational folding are mostly required for cellular activity or signalization in different pathways. Since analytical and diagnostic techniques advanced, proteomics has started to be used in clinical practice more often. In oncology, drugs used to target key proteins like EGFR, VEGF, MAPK, and PI3K and affect their target directly at the protein level not at genomic or transcriptomic level [27]. Phosphorylation status of proteins determines their role in cellular functions and is among the most important issues in oncogenic transformation. In clinical level, use of proteins is more advantageous than other cellular components due to their stable and robust characteristics. At this point, profiling of proteins appears as a useful tool that may help diagnose diseases and determine treatment responses. Most proteomics methodologies are based on quantification and identification of individual proteins *via* Enzyme-Linked Immuno Sorbent Assay (ELISA), Mass Spectroscopy (MS), Nuclear Magnetic Resonance (NMR), and X-ray crystallography. Recently, several studies have used MS technologies to determine biomarkers specific to ovarian and breast cancers [28, 29]. With growing understanding of alterations at the proteomic level, researchers have focused on investigating the differences of individual proteins.

Metabolomics

Metabolomics is a method that emerged after other "omics". Advances in analytical devices and data interpretation have led to rapid development of the metabolic field. NMR, GC-MS and LC-MS techniques are used in metabolomics investigations. These techniques should be evaluated together for the detection of metabolites such as organic acids, amino acids, and lipids in targeted or untargeted metabolomics studies [30].

In case of an identical drug treatment against same cases, examination of the responses may show different individual susceptibility to the disease based on differences in their genetic or metabolic backgrounds. Therefore, it is important to define biomarkers in order to understand the sensitivity of patients against diseases in order to develop personalized treatments.

Specific targeting of a macromolecule or a receptor in cellular milieu is often difficult and off-target effects may lower the efficiency of the therapy. Therefore, directing special cargo-drugs to specific targets is often achieved by NPs. These molecules precisely transport their cargo to the final destination.

Targeted Delivery Through NPs

Personalized medicine is an umbrella term that holds targeted therapy beneath it. As one the leading causes of death worldwide, cancer is widely used in research hoping to reveal new treatment methods. The need for targeted therapy stems from the side effects and limitations of the traditional treatments currently in use. NPs (NPs) can be especially used for targeted delivery of drugs to regions that standard drugs cannot easily reach. In this manner, it is important to aim at disrupted pathways or their components related to the specific disease [2]. Upon specifically targeting cancerous cells, the efficiency of drug delivery is increased while the side effects on healthy cells are diminished [31]. Other than therapeutic drugs; miRNA, siRNA, DNA, plasmids, and oligonucleotides can be carried as well [32].

Targeting the cancer cells with NPs may be *via* passive or active targeting. In passive targeting, tumor properties come to forth. The leaky tumor vasculature and poor lymphatic drainage lead to enhanced permeability and retention (EPR) effect. NPs are naturally carried to tumor core, vasculature and microenvironment, taking advantage of the EPR effect. Smaller NPs are more successful in passive targeting in terms of longer circulation time, higher accumulation in the tumor, and decreased elimination from the system [31]. However, the complexity of the tumor microenvironment is a disadvantage since every tumor is different and so are their EPR effects [33].

Active targeting is used to target specific cancer cells by means of targeting moieties such as monoclonal antibodies, proteins, polymers or aptamers. Certain receptors are specifically overexpressed in cancer cells, which are therefore easily targeted by their specific ligands. Once attached to these receptors, ligands help the accumulation of NPs in the tumor and release their drug content. Specific targeting of any tumor cell receptor is an advantage, however, more research should be done in the area as *in vivo* results are not as successful as *in vitro* results [34].

Types of NPs include; synthetic and natural polymers, inorganic NPs, lipid-based NPs, liposomes, dendrimers, mesoporous silica NPs, nanoshells, quantum dots, metallic NPs, nanohybrids, viral nanocarriers, carbon nanocarriers [32, 33]. They have different abilities for drug loading and can be used in combination with approved traditional treatment methods to carry the advantages one step further. When designing NPs, it is important to consider their biocompatibility, drug encapsulation efficiency, and ability to prevent premature release before reaching their target [33]. Choosing the type of NP is also important as their preparation techniques also vary [32].

Using NPs, it is possible to come up with new treatment formulations. Depending on the type of NP used, induced cytotoxic treatments may be designed, consequently increasing the therapeutic index by promoting fast and efficient treatments. By conjugating a photosensitizer, reactive oxygen species can be produced by radiation to kill cancer cells through photodynamic therapy. In the case of metallic NPs, radiation produces heat using surface plasmon resonance to kill cancer cells with photothermal therapy. In a similar concept to photothermal therapy, magnetic hyperthermia also kills cancer cells with the heat produced by magnetic NPs through magnetic radiation [33].

Drug delivery has multiple challenges that may be overcome with the help of NPs. Uptake of cells is improved, especially in the case of charge-related challenges, when the agent being carried is negatively charged, it slows down the interaction with the cell membrane that is of the same change. Cell-specific ligands may be conjugated to NPs to enhance target specificity. Agents carried are protected from elimination by the macrophages of the reticuloendothelial system (RES) as they are covered and therefore unrecognized and this also prevents immune system activation. Additionally, if the carried agents are nucleic acids, they can escape from nuclease degradation when sheltered by the NP [32].

NPs in cancer therapy have various advantages that count as desirable over the traditional methods. Firstly, their size is ideally small enough to move around the leaky tumor vasculature and big enough not to be eliminated by the system. NP size is one of the important features to be taken into account when considering the success of drug delivery. It should be able to penetrate into the tumor for successful on-target delivery, because the failure of penetration prevents drug delivery into necessary tissue. Studies investigating the effect of particle size on tumor penetrating ability have shown that the two features are inversely proportional. While larger particles accumulate around the blood vessels of the tumor, smaller particles are found throughout the tissue indicating better penetration [35 - 37]. Comparing the time needed for penetration, larger particles also take a while to be distributed within the tumor, but smaller particles can penetrate and distribute within the tumor at ease [38, 39].

NPs can be designed specifically to carry multiple drugs at once for a synergistic effect. In a recent study, biodegradable PGLA (poly(D,L)-lactide-co-glycolide; an FDA-approved polymer) nanofibers able to improve drug delivery across the blood-brain barrier (BBB) were designed [40]. They were loaded with four different drugs (carmustine, irinotecan, cisplatin, and combretastatin) to be released sequentially in the brains of rats with one of the most aggressive primary tumors; glioblastoma multiforme (GBM). After the combined treatment with drugs for different antitumor mechanisms targeting different properties, there was no inflammation developed and drugs were successfully released in high concentrations over the course of two months. Such successful experimental designs indicate that it is possible to target multiple hallmarks of cancer and prevent drug resistance using chemotherapeutic agents with different antitumor activity.

The surface property of NPs is another factor affecting the efficiency of drug delivery. Once introduced into biological fluids, the NP surface is swiftly covered by plasma proteins, in other words, opsonized, to give them an identity to be recognized by the members of the immune system [41]. Additionally, NPs with hydrophobic surfaces tend to aggregate, which also increases the risk of opsonization. Since the formation of this protein corona (PC) may lead to the induction of immune response, surface functionalization is an ideal option to reduce the binding of serum proteins and activation of the immune response [42]. Due to its hydrophilic property, polyethylene glycol (PEG) reduces the chances of NP opsonization and clearance. It is important to ensure the circulation of NP in the bloodstream and increase its half-life in order to increase its stability required for desired targeting [31]. However, studies in the past several years suggest that certain modifications of the PC may open a new window towards therapeutics of different cancers and neurodegenerative diseases [42]. In addition to functionalization, surface properties of NPs can also be used for conjugation of ligands for specific cell types. In the case of cancer, ligands against receptors overexpressed on cancer cells can be conjugated for specific targeting diseased cells and avoiding off-targeting of healthy cells.

Even though a challenging approach, targeted therapy using NPs is a promising novel alternative over traditional cancer treatment methods. NPs owe their efficiency mainly to their small size, surface, and structure properties. Efficiency may be taken even further when these properties are adapted to traditional methods by designing NPs accordingly.

Although the NP approach is promising and has been studied for quite a time, there are issues that should be taken into account. A major drawback of NP research is that studies have mostly focused on *in vitro* models and there is a lack of adequate investigations in *in vivo*. More effort should be given to *in vivo* work to figure out whether the same findings are relevant in both cases.

Stem Cells and Cancer

Stem cells are special populations that are characterized by different properties including self-renewal, migration to tumor site, secretion of soluble cytokines and chemokines, differentiation to numerous cells. Generally, they are classified into two groups; embryonic stem cells (ESCs) and somatic stem cells (SSCs). ESCs are pluripotent cells that have the ability of differentiation to any cell type from all germ layers, unlike those in placenta. Shinya Yamanaka and his team developed induced pluripotent stem cells (iPSCs) from adult cells in 2006 [43]. The potential of these amazing cells has increased the desire to work in this field. Adult stem cells called SSCs are broadly multipotent cells and have the capability of differentiating to all cell types with a specific lineage, such as mesenchymal stem cells (MSCs), hematopoietic stem cells (HSCs), and endothelial progenitor cells (EPCs) [44].

Cancer Treatment with Mesenchymal Stem Cells

Among the type of stem cells, MSCs have the innate tendency for migration to primary or metastatic tumor sites anywhere in the body. Because of their nature, MSCs can practically be manipulated to overexpress proapoptotic molecules to kill tumor cells through apoptosis. Blocking Akt and NF-κB signaling is one of the proapoptotic features of MSCs. Genetic modifications can give new features to MSCs, and then may overcome the restriction of treatment associated with administration of anticancer agents with a short half-life and high toxic effects. Also, MSCs appear to be drug delivery vehicles, which is an important issue of cancer therapy. Recent studies have focused on MSCs as conventional chemoterapeutic agent carriers [45]. However, amount of MSCs need to be given and when and/or where they should be administrated are yet among unanswered questions. Nonetheless, researchers believe that MSCs are the rising stars of the future in personalized cancer therapies.

iPSCs: Return to The Past

Our knowledge about cellular development mechanisms and pluripotency have expanded with the discovery of iPSCs. Thus, this discovery has also allowed improving human-specific diseases and drug screening models. iPSC technology will play a key role in regenerative medicine, as long as the cost and time required for the generation iPSCs reach optimal levels [46].

iPSCs derived from the surgical specimen of a patient with cancer can theoretically be used for generating healthy tissue. In addition, it may be a useful tool to replace damaged tissue in cancer patients. Despite all these promising approaches, iPSC-mediated regenerative therapy has a variety of challenges including vigorously *in vivo* engraftment.

Developing various diseased iPSCs lines makes it easier to investigate human diseases, which are difficult to analyze in animal models. These lines are also a good choice for drug screening and development, disease modelling, cell-based therapy, as well as personalized medicine [47, 48]. The rate of drug failing in clinical trials is pretty high due to adverse effects on heart, liver and central or peripheral nervous systems. Therefore, iPSCs may help us identify drug responses and treatment regimens before clinical trials [49].

FUTURE PERSPECTIVES

Significant improvements have been achieved in nanotheranostics however, cancer is still the second leading cause of death. The nature of many tumors is challenging, and contemporary approaches are required for effective treatment. The translation of nanotheranostics to clinical applications is also challenging. Lack of physiological evidence and extrapolation of animal data to humans need a critical evaluation of biological considerations. The underlying biochemical issues are complex and can only be tested by an *in vivo* system. Only a small portion of *in vitro* theranostic drugs have been found effective *in vivo*.

Nanotheranostics employ nanomaterials to diagnose and treat disease to monitor therapeutic response *in vivo*. Thus, molecular understanding of drug delivery and release as well as optimizing drug response on individual genomic make-up provide deep understanding of the tumor characteristics.

Combining therapy with imaging displays effectiveness of targeted delivery, provides potential applications, and reduces the challenges of nanotheranostic methods for cancer therapy.

CONSENT FOR PUBLICATION

Not applicable.

CONFLICT OF INTEREST

The authors confirm that the contents of this chapter have no conflict of interest.

ACKNOWLEDGEMENTS

Declare none.

REFERENCES

[1]   Hood L, Flores M. A personal view on systems medicine and the emergence of proactive P4 medicine: predictive, preventive, personalized and participatory. N Biotechnol 2012; 29(6): 613-24.
[http://dx.doi.org/10.1016/j.nbt.2012.03.004] [PMID: 22450380]

[2]   Verma M. Personalized medicine and cancer. J Pers Med 2012; 2(1): 1-14.
[http://dx.doi.org/10.3390/jpm2010001] [PMID: 25562699]

[3]   Hood L, Friend SH. Predictive, personalized, preventive, participatory (P4) cancer medicine. Nat Rev Clin Oncol 2011; 8(3): 184-7.
[http://dx.doi.org/10.1038/nrclinonc.2010.227] [PMID: 21364692]

[4]   Blows   WT.   The   Biological   Basis   of   Nursing: Cancer.   London: Routledge 2005.https://www.learner.org
[http://dx.doi.org/10.4324/9780203390559_chapter_1]

[5]   Dreesen O, Brivanlou AH. Signaling pathways in cancer and embryonic stem cells. Stem Cell Rev 2007; 3(1): 7-17.
[http://dx.doi.org/10.1007/s12015-007-0004-8] [PMID: 17873377]

[6]   Febbraio M, Hajjar DP, Silverstein RL. CD36: a class B scavenger receptor involved in angiogenesis, atherosclerosis, inflammation, and lipid metabolism. J Clin Invest 2001; 108(6): 785-91.
[http://dx.doi.org/10.1172/JCI14006] [PMID: 11560944]

[7]   Wang J, Li Y. CD36 tango in cancer: signaling pathways and functions. Theranostics 2019; 9(17): 4893-908.
[http://dx.doi.org/10.7150/thno.36037] [PMID: 31410189]

[8]   James H, Hale S, Otvos B, *et al.* Cancer stem cell-specific scavenger receptor CD36 drives glioblastoma progression. Stem Cells 2015; 32(7): 1746-58.
[http://dx.doi.org/10.1002/stem.1716.Cancer]

[9]   Bitorina AV, Oligschlaeger Y, Shiri-Sverdlov R, Theys J. Low profile high value target: The role of OxLDL in cancer. Biochim Biophys Acta Mol Cell Biol Lipids 2019; 1864(12): 158518.
[http://dx.doi.org/10.1016/j.bbalip.2019.158518] [PMID: 31479734]

[10]   Li C, Zhang J, Wu H, *et al.* Lectin-like oxidized low-density lipoprotein receptor-1 facilitates metastasis of gastric cancer through driving epithelial-mesenchymal transition and PI3K/Akt/GSK3β activation. Sci Rep 2017; 7: 45275.
[http://dx.doi.org/10.1038/srep45275] [PMID: 28345638]

[11]   Scoles DR, Xu X, Wang H, *et al.* Liver X receptor agonist inhibits proliferation of ovarian carcinoma cells stimulated by oxidized low density lipoprotein. Gynecol Oncol 2010; 116(1): 109-16.
[http://dx.doi.org/10.1016/j.ygyno.2009.09.034] [PMID: 19854496]

[12]   Cuomo F, Altucci L, Cobellis G. Autophagy function and dysfunction: Potential drugs as anti-cancer

therapy. Cancers (Basel) 2019; 11(10): E1465.
[http://dx.doi.org/10.3390/cancers11101465] [PMID: 31569540]

[13]   Xie X, Zhang Y, Li F, *et al.* Challenges and opportunities from basic cancer biology for nanomedicine for targeted drug delivery. Curr Cancer Drug Targets 2019; 19(4): 257-76.
[http://dx.doi.org/10.2174/1568009618666180628160211] [PMID: 29956629]

[14]   Xiao Y, Shi K, Qu Y, Chu B, Qian Z. Engineering NPs for targeted delivery of nucleic acid therapeutics in tumor. Mol Ther Methods Clin Dev 2018; 12: 1-18.
[http://dx.doi.org/10.1016/j.omtm.2018.09.002] [PMID: 30364598]

[15]   Lynch HT, Snyder CL, Shaw TG, Heinen CD, Hitchins MP. Milestones of Lynch syndrome: 1895-2015. Nat Rev Cancer 2015; 15(3): 181-94.
[http://dx.doi.org/10.1038/nrc3878] [PMID: 25673086]

[16]   Valencia OM, Samuel SE, Viscusi RK, Riall TS, Neumayer LA, Aziz H. The role of genetic testing in patients with breast cancer: A review. JAMA Surg 2017; 152(6): 589-94.
[http://dx.doi.org/10.1001/jamasurg.2017.0552] [PMID: 28423155]

[17]   Voora D, McLeod HL, Eby C, Gage BF. The pharmacogenetics of coumarin therapy. Pharmacogenomics 2005; 6(5): 503-13.
[http://dx.doi.org/10.2217/14622416.6.5.503] [PMID: 16014000]

[18]   Li W, Wang R, Yan Z, Bai L, Sun Z. High accordance in prognosis prediction of colorectal cancer across independent datasets by multi-gene module expression profiles. PLoS One 2012; 7(3): e33653.
[http://dx.doi.org/10.1371/journal.pone.0033653] [PMID: 22438977]

[19]   Prat A, Ellis MJ, Perou CM. Practical implications of gene-expression-based assays for breast oncologists. Nat Rev Clin Oncol 2011; 9(1): 48-57.
[http://dx.doi.org/10.1038/nrclinonc.2011.178] [PMID: 22143140]

[20]   Botling J, Edlund K, Lohr M, *et al.* Biomarker discovery in non-small cell lung cancer: integrating gene expression profiling, meta-analysis, and tissue microarray validation. Clin Cancer Res 2013; 19(1): 194-204.
[http://dx.doi.org/10.1158/1078-0432.CCR-12-1139] [PMID: 23032747]

[21]   Gokul G, Khosla S. DNA methylation and cancer. Subcell Biochem 2013; 61: 597-625.
[http://dx.doi.org/10.1007/978-94-007-4525-4_26] [PMID: 23150269]

[22]   Audia JE, Campbell RM. Histone modifications and cancer. Cold Spring Harb Perspect Biol 2016; 8(4): a019521.
[http://dx.doi.org/10.1101/cshperspect.a019521] [PMID: 27037415]

[23]   Kohlhapp FJ, Mitra AK, Lengyel E, Peter ME. MicroRNAs as mediators and communicators between cancer cells and the tumor microenvironment. Oncogene 2015; 34(48): 5857-68.
[http://dx.doi.org/10.1038/onc.2015.89] [PMID: 25867073]

[24]   Weller M, Tabatabai G, Kästner B, *et al.* MGMT promoter methylation is a strong prognostic biomarker for benefit from dose-intensified temozolomide rechallenge in progressive glioblastoma: The director trial. Clin Cancer Res 2015; 21(9): 2057-64.
[http://dx.doi.org/10.1158/1078-0432.CCR-14-2737] [PMID: 25655102]

[25]   Tormo E, Ballester S, Adam-Artigues A, *et al.* The miRNA-449 family mediates doxorubicin resistance in triple-negative breast cancer by regulating cell cycle factors. Sci Rep 2019; 9(1): 5316.
[http://dx.doi.org/10.1038/s41598-019-41472-y] [PMID: 30926829]

[26]   Balasubramanian S, Ramos J, Luo W, Sirisawad M, Verner E, Buggy JJ. A novel histone deacetylase 8 (HDAC8)-specific inhibitor PCI-34051 induces apoptosis in T-cell lymphomas. Leukemia 2008; 22(5): 1026-34.
[http://dx.doi.org/10.1038/leu.2008.9] [PMID: 18256683]

[27]   Yaffe MB. The scientific drunk and the lamppost: massive sequencing efforts in cancer discovery and treatment. Sci Signal 2013; 6(269): pe13.

[http://dx.doi.org/10.1126/scisignal.2003684] [PMID: 23550209]

[28]   Swiatly A, Horala A, Matysiak J, Hajduk J, Nowak-Markwitz E, Kokot ZJ. Understanding ovarian cancer: iTRAQ-based proteomics for biomarker discovery. Int J Mol Sci 2018; 19(8): E2240.
       [http://dx.doi.org/10.3390/ijms19082240] [PMID: 30065196]

[29]   Yanovich G, Agmon H, Harel M, Sonnenblick A, Peretz T, Geiger T. Clinical proteomics of breast cancer reveals a novel layer of breast cancer classification. Cancer Res 2018; 78(20): 6001-10.
       [http://dx.doi.org/10.1158/0008-5472.CAN-18-1079] [PMID: 30154156]

[30]   Jacob M, Lopata AL, Dasouki M, Abdel Rahman AM. Metabolomics toward personalized medicine. Mass Spectrom Rev 2019; 38(3): 221-38.
       [http://dx.doi.org/10.1002/mas.21548] [PMID: 29073341]

[31]   Raj S, Khurana S, Choudhari R, *et al.* Specific targeting cancer cells with NPs and drug delivery in cancer therapy. Semin Cancer Biol 2019.; S1044-579X(19): 30216-0.
       [http://dx.doi.org/10.1016/j.semcancer.2019.11.002] [PMID: 31715247]

[32]   Lee SWL, Paoletti C, Campisi M, *et al.* MicroRNA delivery through NPs. J Control Release 2019; 313: 80-95.
       [http://dx.doi.org/10.1016/j.jconrel.2019.10.007] [PMID: 31622695]

[33]   VanDyke D, Kyriacopulos P, Yassini B, *et al.* NP based combination treatments for targeting multiple hallmarks of cancer. Int J Nano Stud Technol 2016; 1-18.
       [http://dx.doi.org/10.19070/2167-8685-SI04001]

[34]   Bertrand N, Wu J, Xu X, Kamaly N, Farokhzad OC. Cancer nanotechnology: the impact of passive and active targeting in the era of modern cancer biology. Adv Drug Deliv Rev 2014; 66: 2-25.
       [http://dx.doi.org/10.1016/j.addr.2013.11.009] [PMID: 24270007]

[35]   Wang CE, Stayton PS, Pun SH, Convertine AJ. Polymer nanostructures synthesized by controlled living polymerization for tumor-targeted drug delivery. J Control Release 2015; 219: 345-54.
       [http://dx.doi.org/10.1016/j.jconrel.2015.08.054] [PMID: 26342661]

[36]   Perry JL, Reuter KG, Luft JC, Pecot CV, Zamboni W, DeSimone JM. Mediating passive tumor accumulation through particle size, tumor type, and location. Nano Lett 2017; 17(5): 2879-86.
       [http://dx.doi.org/10.1021/acs.nanolett.7b00021] [PMID: 28287740]

[37]   Vlashi E, Kelderhouse LE, Sturgis JE, Low PS. Effect of folate-targeted NP size on their rates of penetration into solid tumors. ACS Nano 2013; 7(10): 8573-82.
       [http://dx.doi.org/10.1021/nn402644g] [PMID: 24020507]

[38]   Mikhail AS, Eetezadi S, Ekdawi SN, Stewart J, Allen C. Image-based analysis of the size- and time-dependent penetration of polymeric micelles in multicellular tumor spheroids and tumor xenografts. Int J Pharm 2014; 464(1-2): 168-77.
       [http://dx.doi.org/10.1016/j.ijpharm.2014.01.010] [PMID: 24440400]

[39]   Gray BP, McGuire MJ, Brown KC. A liposomal drug platform overrides peptide ligand targeting to a cancer biomarker, irrespective of ligand affinity or density. PLoS One 2013; 8(8): e72938.
       [http://dx.doi.org/10.1371/journal.pone.0072938] [PMID: 24009717]

[40]   Tseng YY, Yang TC, Wang YC, *et al.* Targeted concurrent and sequential delivery of chemotherapeutic and antiangiogenic agents to the brain by using drug-loaded nanofibrous membranes. Int J Nanomed 2017; 12: 1265-76.
       [http://dx.doi.org/10.2147/IJN.S124593] [PMID: 28243088]

[41]   Barbero F, Russo L, Vitali M, *et al.* Formation of the protein corona: The interface between NPs and the immune system. Semin Immunol 2017; 34: 52-60.
       [http://dx.doi.org/10.1016/j.smim.2017.10.001] [PMID: 29066063]

[42]   Nierenberg D, Khaled AR, Flores O. Formation of a protein corona influences the biological identity of nanomaterials. Rep Pract Oncol Radiother 2018; 23(4): 300-8.
       [http://dx.doi.org/10.1016/j.rpor.2018.05.005] [PMID: 30100819]

[43]   Takahashi K, Yamanaka S. Induction of pluripotent stem cells from mouse embryonic and adult fibroblast cultures by defined factors. Cell 2006; 126(4): 663-76.
[http://dx.doi.org/10.1016/j.cell.2006.07.024] [PMID: 16904174]

[44]   Zakrzewski W, Dobrzyński M, Szymonowicz M, Rybak Z. Stem cells: past, present, and future. Stem Cell Res Ther 2019; 10(1): 68.
[http://dx.doi.org/10.1186/s13287-019-1165-5] [PMID: 30808416]

[45]   Layek B, Sadhukha T, Panyam J, Prabha S. Nano-engineered mesenchymal stem cells increase therapeutic efficacy of anticancer drug through true active tumor targeting. Mol Cancer Ther 2018; 17(6): 1196-206.
[http://dx.doi.org/10.1158/1535-7163.MCT-17-0682] [PMID: 29592881]

[46]   Rathod R, Surendran H, Battu R, Desai J, Pal R. Induced pluripotent stem cells (iPSC)-derived retinal cells in disease modeling and regenerative medicine. J Chem Neuroanat 2019; 95: 81-8.
[http://dx.doi.org/10.1016/j.jchemneu.2018.02.002] [PMID: 29448001]

[47]   Lang C, Campbell KR, Ryan BJ, *et al.* Single-cell sequencing of iPSC-dopamine neurons reconstructs disease progression and identifies HDAC4 as a regulator of parkinson cell phenotypes. Cell Stem Cell 2019; 24(1): 93-106.e6.
[http://dx.doi.org/10.1016/j.stem.2018.10.023] [PMID: 30503143]

[48]   Gorecka J, Kostiuk V, Fereydooni A, *et al.* The potential and limitations of induced pluripotent stem cells to achieve wound healing. Stem Cell Res Ther 2019; 10(1): 87.
[http://dx.doi.org/10.1186/s13287-019-1185-1] [PMID: 30867069]

[49]   Edwards IR, Aronson JK. Adverse drug reactions: Definitions, diagnosis, and management. Lancet 2000; 356(9237): 1255-9.
[http://dx.doi.org/10.1016/S0140-6736(00)02799-9] [PMID: 11072960]

CHAPTER 2

Tumor Microenvironment: A Critical Determinant in Regulating Tumor Progression and Metastasis

Raghda Ashraf Soliman[1], Rana Ahmed Youness[1,*] and **Mohamed Zakaria Gad[2,*]**

[1] *Pharmaceutical Biology Department, Faculty of Pharmacy and Biotechnology, German University in Cairo, 11835, Cairo, Egypt*

[2] *Biochemistry Department, Faculty of Pharmacy and Biotechnology, German University in Cairo, 11835, Cairo, Egypt*

Abstract: The fate of cancer cells is predicted not only by its intrinsic oncogenic engines, but also by its surrounding milieu. Beyond the tumor margin at the tumor microenvironment (TME), there is an orchestra of immune cells and soluble mediators known as the cellular and non-cellular components of TME that shape the tumor architecture. Several reports have focused on immune cells influencing the cellular components of the TME, therefore the main focus of our chapter will be the non-cellular components of TME. The non-cellular components of TME include cytokines, chemokines, growth factors, inflammatory and extra-cellular matrix remodeling enzymes that are released by the tumor cells or associated immune cells in the TME. These soluble mediators outline the progression of the disease by mediating the communication taking place between the tumor cell itself and its surrounding. Considering that TME is a critical determinant in unraveling the complexity of cancer cells, thus, zooming in at the TME would definitely help us pave the road for new combinatory immuno-oncological interventions incorporating the TME in their mechanism of action and thus lowering the chances of relapse rates among cancer patients.

Keywords: Angiogenesis, Angiogenic switch, Cancer Associated Fibroblasts (CAF), Cytokines, Chemokines, Extracellular Matrix (ECM), Growth factors (GFs), Hypoxia, Hypoxia inducing Factor-1 (HIF-1), Inflammation, Immune surveillance, Remodeling enzymes, Tumor microenvironment (TME), Tumor Infiltrating Lymphocytes (TILs), T cell exhaustion, Tumor associated Macrophages (TAMs).

---

* **Corresponding authors Dr. Rana Ahmed Youness:** Pharmaceutical Biology Department, Faculty of Pharmacy and Biotechnology, German University in Cairo, 11835, Cairo, Egypt; E-mails: rana.ahmed-youness@guc.edu.eg; rana.youness21@gmail.com, **Prof. Mohamed Zakaria Gad:** Biochemistry Department, Faculty of Pharmacy and Biotechnology, German University in Cairo, 11835, Cairo, Egypt; Tel: 002-01272222695; Fax: +202-2-2759 0711; E-mail: Mohamed.gad@guc.edu.eg

THE TUMOR MICROENVIRONMENT

Cancer is not just abnormal cells that continue to grow and metastasize, it is a complex tissue made up of tumor cells and their surrounding stroma [1]. These tumor cells can communicate with the cellular and non-cellular components in their surroundings. This is referred to as the tumor microenvironment (TME) [2]. TME can modulate the tumor's aggressiveness, rate of growth, immune recognition and metastatic properties [3].

The cellular components of the TME have been extensively studied. They mainly include T-lymphocytes [4, 5], $CD4^+$ T cells [6, 7], $CD8^+$ T cells [8, 9], regulatory T cells (Tregs) [10], B-lymphocytes, natural Killer (NK) cells [11], mesenchymal stem cells (MSCs) [12], tumor-associated-macrophages (TAMs) [13, 14], myeloid derived suppressor cells (MDSCs) [15 - 17], tumor-associated neutrophils (TANs) [18, 19], and terminally differentiated myeloid dendritic cells (DCs) [20], pericytes [21], adipocytes [22, 23], and cancer associated fibroblastic cells (CAFs) [24, 25] as shown in Fig. (**1**). The non-cellular TME components include cytokines, chemokines, growth factors, inflammatory and extracellular matrix remodeling enzymes; all of which play role in the communication taking place between the tumor itself and its surroundings [26]. In this chapter, we will be mainly discussing the cellular and non-cellular components of TME and their integrated interplay to dictate the fate of tumor cells. Nonetheless, we will shed light on the potential role of TME in the immune-therapeutic equation and its consideration in the new combinatory therapeutic intervention evading the immuno-oncology market.

CELLULAR COMPONENTS OF THE TME

The immune setting within the TME significantly determines cancer fate. A strong lymphocytic infiltration has been paradoxically reported to be associated with good or poor clinical outcomes in different human tumors depending on the type of immune cells infiltrating the TME [27 - 29].

Tumor Infiltrating Lymphocytes

The term tumor-infiltrating lymphocytes (TILs) was first made up by Wallace Clark in 1969 and later defined operationally as a lymphocyte that has migrated from bloodstream towards tumor cells. More recently, the term TILs has been used to describe a variety of tumor-infiltrating cells including T cells, B cells, macrophages, DCs, NK cells, and MDSCs [30].

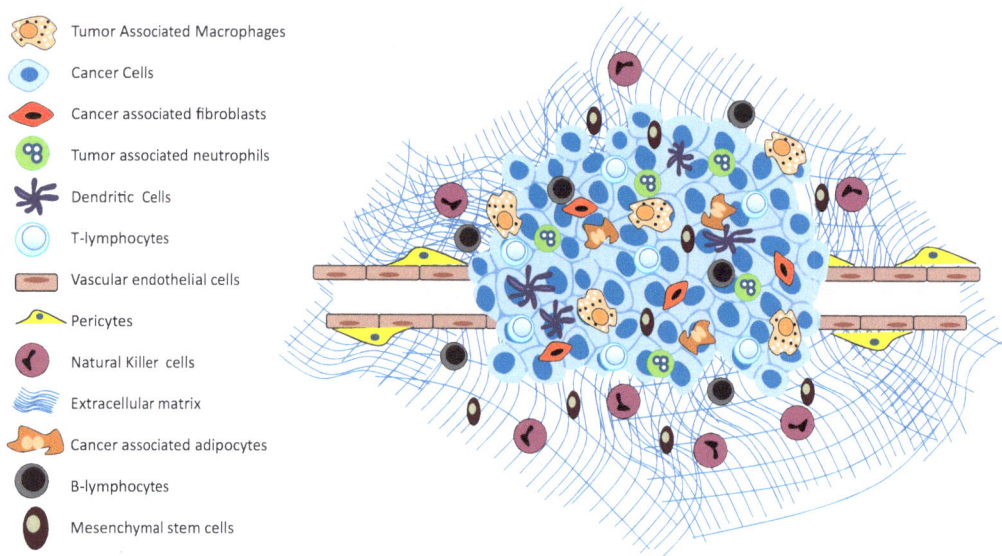

Fig. (1). Cellular components of the tumor microenvironment: Tumor Associated Macrophages (TAMs), Cancer Associated Fibroblasts (CAFs), Tumor Associated Neutrophils (TANs), Dentritic Cells (DCs), T-lymphocytes, Vascular endothelial cells, pericytes, Natural Killer cels (NKs), Cancer associated adipocytes, B-lymphocytes, Mesenchymal Stem Cells (MSCs) and Extracellular matrix of the tumor.

T-lymphocytes

T cells are divided into two types according to their clusters of differentiation (CD); $CD4^+$ T (helper T cells, Th) and $CD8^+$ T (cytotoxic T cells, Tc) cells. $CD4^+$ cells further compromise subtypes besides the classical T-helper 1 (Th1) and T-helper 2 (Th2) cells [31, 32]. These include T-helper 17 (Th17), follicular helper T cell (Tfh), induced T-regulatory cells (iTreg), and the regulatory type 1 cells (Tr1) as well as the potentially distinct T-helper 9 (Th9) [33 - 35]. This differentiation is due to the complex cytokine signaling network, transcription factors, and epigenetic alterations [36]. Tumors have the ability to suppress T cells once they migrate into the tumor margin or infiltrate a tumor tissue where they encounter the TME [37]. Three signals are required for T cell activation. At the tumor-immune synapse, first, the MHC-peptide complex is recognized by T cell receptor. Then, the pairing of co-stimulatory or co-inhibitory molecules occurs, and finally, proper soluble mediators are produced. Of these signals, the pairing step to co-inhibitory/stimulatory molecules is crucial in mounting the cytokine profile responsible for the differentiation of lymphocytes into either activator or inhibitor phenotypes. In normal scenarios, co-inhibitory molecules such as PD-1 and CTLA-4 inhibit inflammation and prevent the unfortunate increase of immune system responses and tissue damage. However, in cancer, an excessive rise of co-inhibitory signals takes place wearying immune responses and resulting in T cells exhaustion. This exhaustion enhances the expression of the inhibitory receptors PD-1 and CTLA-4 and reduces the production of granzyme B and the stimulatory cytokines IL-2, IFN-γ, and TNF-α [38, 39]. Although T lymphocytes can have an anti-tumor effects, the presence of immune suppressive agents at the TME leads to repeated activation of T cells, which causes T cells to acquire more inhibitory receptors, along with reduced proliferation, and decreased cytokine production. Thus, TME provides the optimum conditions for T cells to become exhausted as well as being able to maintain this state during cancer progression. Therefore, blocking such inhibitory receptors with specific antibodies such as PD-1 and CTLA-4 inhibitors (Immune-checkpoint blockades) may re-energize the antitumor responses of exhausted T cells.

B-lymphocytes

In addition to the role of T cells in shaping the tumor immunosurveillance [40], an emerging role for B cells is recently being highlighted [41]. B cells have immunosuppressive and/or regulatory functions that can modulate anti-tumor immune responses [42]. They are classically known to positively modulate immune responses and inflammation through antibody production, T cell activation, and proliferation through antigen presentation [43]. The presence of B cells varies according to tumor status. They could be found in the invasive margins, but not as much as in the lymphoid structures next to the TME or the drainage lymphatic system. B cell infiltration at TME is considered a good prognostic marker in ovarian cancer and some breast cancer subtypes [44, 45]. The role of B cells at TME extends beyond provoking the humoral immune responses. They have the capacity to recognize antigens, regulate antigen processing and presentation, and mount and modulate T cell and innate immune responses. Furthermore, through antibody production and the formation of antigen–antibody complexes, B cells could possibly influence all immune cell types expressing Fc receptors (DCs, NK cells, and MDSCs) [46]. However, anti-tumor effects of B cells were found to be particularly exerted through the enhancement of cytotoxic T cell activity, exertion of a direct tumoricidal effect by secretion of granzyme B, or indirectly through antibody-dependent mechanisms [46]. Yet, one of the potential soldiers downstream of the B cells is the release of several cytokines, such as IFN-γ, which could polarize T cells towards a Th1 or Th2 response. Still, the characteristics that differentiate tumor promoting and tumor suppressive effects of B cells remain largely unknown.

Natural Killer (NK) Cells

NK cells are one of the fundamental components of TME that have potent tumoricidal effects. However, some tumor promoting immune cells have been demonstrated to directly suppress NK cells. In such context, Tregs from patients with gastrointestinal sarcoma (GIST) have been shown to inhibit NK cells through membrane-bound TGF-β [47, 48]. Melanoma-derived primary cell lines were also shown to inhibit the expression of NKp30, NKp44, and NKG2D *in vitro*, which are activating receptors on NK cells, thus preventing NK cells from identifying and killing tumor cells [49].

Myeloid Derived Suppressor Cells (MDSCs)

The irregular differentiation and function of myeloid cells at the TME is considered to be one of the cancer hallmarks. The accumulation of immature, pathologically activated MDSC with potent immunosuppressive activity supports tumor development. MDSCs can play a role in remodeling the tumor microenvironment [50, 51], promoting invasion, angiogenesis, tumor cell survival and metastasis that have been previously reviewed in [52]. MDSCs have been shown to produce VEGF and MMP9, which are mediators of neo-angiogenesis and tissue invasion at the tumor site [53 - 55]. Expression of these mediators has been linked to MDSC-mediated metastasis and is independent of their immunosuppressive capacity [56].

Tumor Associated Macrophages (TAMs)

Macrophages at TME can constitute up to 50% of all immune cell infiltrates [14, 57]. TAMs have a dynamic role from early carcinogenesis to tumor progression till metastasis [4]. Even though TAMs are considered to be anti-tumor in the early stages of cancer, once the tumor is established; they switch to a pro-tumoral phenotype [58]. This pro-tumoral activity is suggested to be due to acquired properties of M2-like phagocytic population and phenotypes. This includes the promotion of angiogenesis, suppression of antitumor immunity, tumor growth, and remodeling of tissues [59]. TAMs are considered to be essential components of the immune cell infiltrates responsible for malignant cell invasion, migration, and metastases [60]. Moreover, they release inhibitory cytokines such as IL-10, reactive oxygen species or prostaglandins inhibiting the lymphocyte functions [61, 62].

Tumor Associated Neutrophils (TANs)

Neutrophils account for about 60% of all leukocytes. They are the first line of defense at the site of infection or inflammation. Contrary to its recognized properties of activating immunity and inducing tissue damage in infections, it acts as immunosuppressive cells in tumors [63]. In early cancer stages, TANs are found at the periphery of the tumor and are suggested to be more cytotoxic toward tumor cells, producing higher levels of TNF-α, NO, and H_2O_2. However, once tumors are established, these actions become downregulated and TANs acquire more protumorigenic phenotype and are scattered among tumor cells [64].

Dendritic Cells (DCs)

DCs are subset of cells at TME which can alter their role from being immunostimulatory to immunosuppressive at different stages of cancer progression [65]. DCs express innate inflammatory cytokines, such as IL-1, IL-12 and IL-23 that promote the response of CD4+ T cells and cytotoxic T lymphocyte to secrete IFN-γ [66]. Not surprisingly, due to the complexity of phenotype as well as the methods of identification, DC infiltration has been reported to be associated with both good and poor prognosis in different tumor types. While not yet clear what specifically induces these phenotypic shifts, release of cytokines or other factors into the TME are likely to be involved [67].

Adipocytes

Adipocytes are fat cells found in the TME. They secrete adipokines, which recruit malignant cells and promote their growth by providing fatty acids as fuel for them [68]. Moreover, adipocytes secrete different cytokines, chemokines, and hormone-like factors [69, 70], which can contribute to tumor initiation.

Cancer Associated Fibroblasts (CAFs)

A sub-population of fibroblasts in cancer with a myofibroblastic phenotype is known as cancer-associated fibroblasts (CAFs) [71 - 73]. During the physiological wound repair process, myofibroblasts are only transiently present [74]. Unlike wound repair, CAFs at the site of a tumor remain activated after the initial insult has regressed. These activated CAFs can lead to cancer progression and metastasis through their angiogenesis and metastatic ability compared to normal fibroblasts [75].

Non-cellular Components

The second main group in TME is the non-cellular components. These including several soluble mediators are released by either the tumor cells or the associated immune cells at the tumor-immune synapse orchestrating the crosstalk within TME. This crosstalk is crucial in determining the fate of tumor cell proliferation, invasion, and metastasis. As mentioned earlier, non-cellular components include cytokines, chemokines, growth-factors, inflammatory and remodeling enzymes, which are summarized in Table **1** and will be separately discussed below.

Table 1. Non-cellular components at the Tumor Microenvironment (TME).

Non-cellular Components at the TME	Function	References
IL-1	• IL-1α is involved in the suppression of keratinocyte differentiation markers, leading to neoplastic transformation in a cell-autonomous manner.	[123]
I-2	• Promotes Cytotoxic T-cells and NK cell proliferation.	[124]
IL-4	• Suppresses tumor immunity, and supports the generation of immunosuppressive cells as TAMs and MDSCs. • Promotes tumor growth by supporting angiogenesis and creating an immunosuppressive environment that inhibits lytic activity of Cytotoxic T cells and NK cells. • In the TME of breast cancer, IL-4 was found to induce cancer cell growth, survival and metastasis mediated by MAPK signaling pathway.	[125 - 128]
IL-6	• A pro-inflammatory cytokine known to alter stromal cell function, migration, and EMT in the tumor microenvironment. • IL-6 not only activates inflammation but also controls a number of pro-cancer activities like progression, malignancy and anti-death signaling pathways. • IL-6 can act as a protective shield against DNA damage by inducing pro-cancer signaling repair pathways. • IL-6 also attenuates the surface expression level of MHC class II and IL-12 production of human dendritic cells and suppress IFNγ-production from Th cells.	[129 - 131]
IL-8	• IL-8 produces self- and cross-reinforced inflammatory microenvironment responsible for aggressive phenotypes to a luminal breast cancer cell line.	[132]
IL-10	• IL-10 is secreted by Tumor cells and TAMs. • IL-10 is considered a growth factor required in signaling of the inflammatory response and invasion of immune cells, acts differently in the TME. It is found to specifically trigger cancer progression and tumor maintenance. • IL-10 has been considered as a target to enhance antitumor immunity, as It down-regulates MHC affecting antigen-presenting cells and co-stimulatory molecules.t diminishes the expression of TH1 cytokines like IFN-γ, and induces Tregs. • The anti-inflammatory cytokine IL-10 may also contribute to tumor growth. In a mouse model of melanoma, tumors overexpressing IL-10 present a higher tumor growth mediated by an increase in tumor cell proliferation, angiogenesis, and immune evasion.	[133 - 135]
IL-12	• Induce Th1-type response and a potent CTL activity mediated mainly by CD8+ T cells; IL-12 is able to induce IFN- γ release from effector cells.	[136]
IL-13	• Mediate the invasion and metastasis in different cancer types.	[137, 138]

(Table 1) cont.....

Non-cellular Components at the TME	Function	References
IL-15	• IL-15 is a cytokine that is constitutively expressed in multiple tissues by many cell types to maintain the normal homeostasis of T cells and NK cells. • IL-15 also promotes antitumor functions within the TME.	[139 - 142]
IL-17	• IL-17C promotes the recruitment of neutrophils, tumor-associated inflammation and tumor proliferation and growth.	[143]
IL-21	• Induces Tregs function, induces M1 polarization. (M1 is the classically activated macrophages, pro-inflammatory type).	[144, 145]
IL-22	• IL-22 directly stimulate endothelial cell proliferation, survival and migration.	[146]
IL-23	• Promotes suppression of immune system by decreasing the permeation of CD4+ T cells and CD8+ T cells into tumor tissues.	[147]
IL-33	• Promotes tumor growth by acting as a nuclear factor to activate NF-κB and MAPK signaling pathways that enhance proliferation. • Promote cancer angiogenesis and vasopermeability independent of VEGF, possibly by increasing endothelial cell proliferation, migration, or tubular network formation. • IL-33 is highly involved in several cancers where this cytokine exerts protumorigenic and antitumorigenic functions up to the environment.	[148 - 151] [25]
IL-35	• IL-35 inhibits the normal function of immune cells like neutrophils, leading to failure of immunotherapy.	[152]
TNF-α	• This cytokine can act as both a tumor inhibitor by stimulating the activity or number of these immune suppressor cells, and inhibition of angiogenesis. And protumor by acting as a promoter of premetastatic niche formation in tumors.	[153, 154]
Type I IFNs (IFN-α and IFN-β) Type I IFNs (IFN-γ)	• IFN-I is contributed to the recruitment of M1 macrophages, production of CTL, and inhibition of Tregs functioning within the TME. • IFN-γ is a proinflammatory cytokine that its function is for inhibition of angiogenesis in cancer cells.	[10, 153, 155, 156]

(Table 1) cont.....

Non-cellular Components at the TME	Function	References
CXCL12 and CCL20 CCR6 CCR4 and CCL22 CCL2	• High levels of CXCL12 (also known as SDF1; the ligand for CXCR4) and CC-chemokine ligand 20 (CCL20; the ligand for CCR6 are found in human tumor microenvironments. This chemokine profile may facilitate the trafficking of TH17 cells into tumors. • TH22 cells are found in the microenvironment of several types of human cancer, including colon cancer, pancreatic cancer and hepatocellular carcinoma. These cells express CCR6, migrate towards the CCR6 ligand CCL20 in the colon cancer microenvironment, and have been shown to promote and support tumorigenesis. • Another way in which chemokines may promote tumorigenesis is by mediating the recruitment of regulatory T (Treg) cells into the tumor microenvironment. Treg cells express CCR4 and are recruited into the tumor micro environment in response to CCL22, which is produced mainly by macrophages and tumor cells. • Most NKT cells express non-lymphoid-homing or inflammation-related chemokine receptors including CCR2, CCR5 and CXCR3. CCL2 mediates the trafficking of type I NKT cells into neuroblastomas. • . NKT cell trafficking into other types of tumor is poorly studied High levels of tumor-infiltrating B cells are associated with a survival advantage in breast cancer.	[157 - 159] [160 - 163] [164] [165 - 167] [168]
VEGF-A	• Vascular endothelial growth factor-A (VEGF-A) is an important biomarker which plays crucial role in angiogenesis during tumor progression by binding to its receptors (VEGFR1 and VEGFR2) and is found to be over-expressed in different neoplastic diseases.	[169, 170].
MMP-2	• MMP2 promotes invasion and metastasis *via* ECM degradation.	[171]
MMP28	• MMPs are a family of structurally related zinc dependent endopeptidases collectively capable of degrading almost all components of extracellular matrix. MMPs are important not only in normal, physiological and biological processes such as embryogenesis, normal tissue remodelling, wound healing and angiogenesis but also in diseases such as arthritis, cancer& tissue ulceration. • MMP28 causes the proteolytic activation of TGF $-\beta$ which is a powerful inducer of EMT. Epithelial mesenchymal transition is a process in which epithelial cells change from epithelial phenotype to mesenchymal phenotype leading to loss of epithelial integrity, increased migration, invasion and ultimately metastasis.	[172] [173, 174]

Cytokines

As a fundamental part of TME, cytokines can act as pro-inflammatory, anti-inflammatory or both according to their settings and conditions [76]. The initiation and progression of inflammation and cancer are aggravated by dysregulated expression of cytokines controlling diverse cellular phenotypes including differentiation, apoptosis, angiogenesis, and cell invasiveness [77] as shown in Table **1**. Significant inflammation always accompanies tumor growth; thus, an increase in pro-inflammatory cytokine levels is usually noticed in different cancer types [76].

Cytokines are categorized into multiple families, based on differences in their structure, receptors, and signaling mechanisms. Types include type I (hematopoietic family) and type II (interferon family) cytokines, tumor necrosis factor (TNF) family, interleukins, stem cell factor/receptor tyrosine kinase (STF/RTK) cytokines, transforming growth factor-β (TGF-β) family, and a seventh group, known as chemokines, that form a separate family and bind seven transmembrane domain receptors as shown in Fig. (**2**) [78, 79].

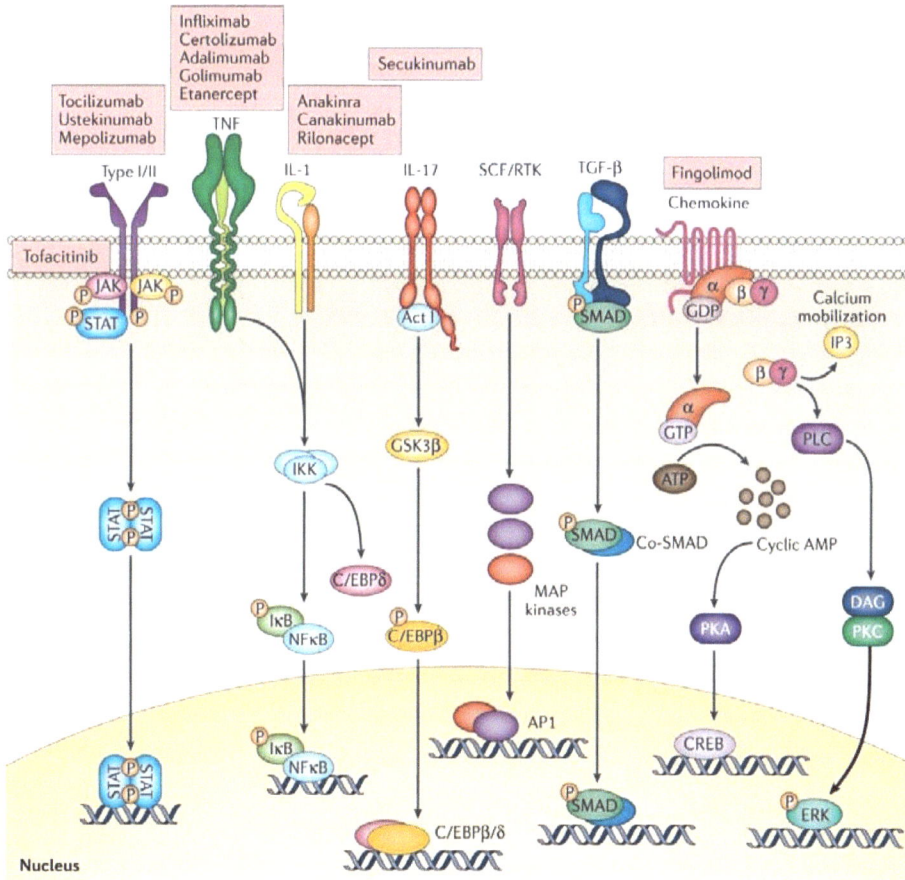

Nature Reviews | Rheumatology

Fig. (2). Cytokines are grouped into super families based on shared structural elements of the receptors they bind [79].

Type I cytokine, also known as the hematopoietin, constitute the largest group among the cytokine family [80, 81]. It includes IL-2 receptor-γ subunit. Cytokines include IL-2, IL-4, IL-7, IL-9, IL-15, and IL-21. Many γc cytokines have also been implicated in diverse autoimmune diseases. IL-2 is the prototypic T cell growth factor and has both pro-inflammatory and anti-inflammatory effects. This cytokine is important for effector T cells, upregulating production of other cytokines and augmenting the cytolytic activity of CD8+ T cells and NK cells [82].

Type II cytokines includes all three IFNs types: type I, II, and III. Type I IFN contains two subtypes; IFN-α and IFN-β [83] mainly expressed by innate immune cells [84]. IFN-ω and IFN-τ remain poorly characterized [85, 86]. Type II IFN contains IFN-γ, known for its antiviral activity by activated immune cells [87, 88]. Type III IFNs (also called IFN-λ/interleukin IL-28 and IL-29) are the least characterized, they are restricted in their tissue distribution and act at epithelial surfaces [89, 90]. The family also includes IL-10, IL-19, IL-20, IL-22, IL-24, IL-26 as with IL-10 being the main member [91 - 97].

TNF family diverse functions are executed *via* signaling through two TNF receptors (TNFR) which mediate different cell activities. TNFR1 and TNFR2 are expressed by immune cells. TNFR2 is also expressed by endothelial cells. TNF induces programmed cell death *via* TNFR1 to activate inflammatory signals. TNFR1 possesses a critical death domain in the cytoplasmic tail, while TNFR2 does not [98].

The Interleukin-1 (IL- 1) family plays a central role in the modulation of innate immunity and inflammation [99, 100]. The family contains (IL-1α, IL-1β, IL-18, IL-33, one anti-inflammatory cytokine (IL-37), and the IL-36 subfamily which is comprised of IL-36α, IL-36β, IL-36γ as well as the IL-36 Receptor antagonist (IL-36Ra) [101]. The IL-1 family members signal through Toll/IL-1 receptor (TIR) domain [99]. Disturbances in the homeostasis of the IL-1 cytokines usually promotes a wide range of inflammatory diseases [102].

IL-17 family, contains five members, IL-17 A-E, all of which are single-pass transmembrane receptors with conserved structural features [103]. Most IL-17 cytokine signals occur through heterodimeric receptors composed of a common IL-17RA chain and a second chain that determines ligand or signaling specificity. The second receptor chains are as follows: IL-17RC for IL-17A and IL-17F [104], IL-17RB for IL-17E [105] and IL-17RE for IL-17C [106].

Chemokines as mentioned are known for their effect on directing the movement of circulating leukocytes to the site of inflammation or injury [107]. They activate the production and secretion of inflammatory mediators [108]. There are various biochemical and cellular mechanisms by which the interactions between chemokines and their receptors are regulated. These include selective and competitive binding interactions, genetic polymorphisms, messenger RNA splice variation, variation of expression, degradation, and localization, downregulation by atypical receptors, interactions with cel-surface glycosaminoglycans, posttranslational modifications, oligomerization, alternative signaling responses, and binding to natural or pharmacological inhibitors [109].

Chemokines

Chemokines are small chemotactic proteins that mediate lymphoid tissue development and immune cell trafficking [110, 111]. Chemokines are further subdivided into four main classes depending on the location of the first two cysteine (C) residues in their protein sequence: CC chemokines, CXC-chemokines, C-chemokines and. CX3C-chemokines [111]. Both chemokines and chemokine receptors are produced by TME cells, as well as by tumor cells themselves and may induce proliferation and/or survival of tumor cells, thereby acting as paracrine or autocrine stimulators of tumor growth [112] as shown in Table **1**.

Growth Factors

Growth factors (GFs) are essential for clonal expansion, as they increase susceptibility of cells to oncogenic mutations. Many cancer cells synthesize their own GFs, making it a way to promote cancer progression [113, 114] as shown in Table **1**. For example, insulin-like growth factor-1 receptor (IGF-1R), is ubiquitously expressed in different types of cancer, and is involved in diverse processes including mitogenesis, cell survival and differentiation. Dysregulation of GFs have also been reported and is involved in tumorigenesis. A study has highlighted for the first time that the down-regulation of IGF-1 in NK cells of HCC patients could be one of the factors associated with the impaired functions of those NK cells [115]. This interestingly links both cellular and non-cellular components of TME and their involvement in the disease progression.

ECM Remodeling Enzymes

ECM remodeling enzymes have been linked in many studies as a key factor in promoting cancer, such as prostate cancer [116], melanoma [117], cervical cancer [118], breast cancer [119], colon cancer [120], ovarian cancer [121]. The ECM is important in maintaining the architecture of the stroma without which epithelial mesenchymal transition occurs, a hallmark in cancer progression [122] as shown in Table **1**.

TME and Therapy

It has become obligatory in the clinical setting to destroy cancer cells by targeting TME. The complexity of the cellular and non-cellular components of the tumor surroundings, and their similarity with normal tissue remains a challenge in the development of a definite therapeutic approach. Despite the increased number of studies and better understanding of cancer development and its hallmarks, current therapies are still not fully efficient to fight off cancer.

Tumor infiltrates at the TME is composed of a variety of immune and inflammatory cells, blood endothelial cells and lymphatic endothelial cells, that lead to (lymph) angiogenic switch as described in this book chapter [75, 175]. Acknowledging the importance of the tumor microenvironment in cancer progression has led to a shift from a tumor-centered approach to a tumor-local-environment view in which cancer evolution and metastasis take place. One feature of the TME is that a slight change in only one component may cause a dramatic reorganization of the whole system. Therefore, interference with TME elements can give an opportunity to neutralize cancer progression and give hope for a better therapy outcome for cancer patients. Currently, several therapeutic interventions are inspired by such concept and are targeting several TME hallmarks as elaborated below.

Targeting Tumor Microenvironment

Cancer cells are able to escape from the immune surveillance mechanisms and settle down deep within normal tissues and create their unique permissive settings. Immune surveillance is the ability of immune system to identify cancerous and/or pre-cancerous cells and eliminate them before they cause harm. Despite the tumor immune surveillance, tumors do develop in the presence of a functioning immune system [176]. Autocrine and paracrine communications between TME cellular components induce TME hypoxia, inflammation, angiogenesis, infiltration and residing of more TILs, and remodeling of ECM which will be discussed below [1].

Targeting TME Hypoxia

For a tumor cell to quickly proliferate, a high amount of oxygen is required. This cannot be sustained by the surrounding blood supply; therefore, hypoxia takes place. The partial oxygen pressure within the TME is generally lower compared to normal tissues. In addition, the TME may experience two types of low oxygenation events, chronic and acute/cycling hypoxia [177, 178]. This response to low oxygen pressure levels includes regulation of genes involved in glucose metabolism, cell proliferation, angiogenesis, macrophage polarization into tumor-associated macrophages (TAM), and metastasis [179, 180]. Hypoxia triggers a series of cellular responses to counteract the oxygen deficit experienced by the cell, mainly coordinated by the transcriptional factor hypoxia-induced factor-1 (HIF-1) [181]. Several compounds and therapies were designed to tackle HIF-1 or its targets to avoid tumor progression [182, 183].

Targeting Inflammation

Another commonly recognized cancer trait is chronic inflammation involved in cancer expansion. Pre-clinical evidence supports the use of anti-inflammatory drugs for cancer therapy. Inflammation inhibitors are aimed to inhibit signal transducers and transcription factors that mediate tumor growth and survival, or inhibit tumor promoting chemokines and cytokines that promote tumor infiltration by inflammatory cells such as interleukin 1 (IL-1), IL-6, tumor necrosis factor alpha, TNFα, or receptor antagonists targeting C-C chemokine receptor types 2 and 4 and C-X-C chemokine receptor type 4, or depletes immune and inflammatory cells of the tumor infiltrate such as MDSCs and macrophages that promote tumor development [175, 184].

Targeting Angiogenesis

Tumor progression and survival depends on nutrients and oxygen provided by the formation of new blood vessels. This vascularized state is called the "angiogenic switch", and is dependent on cancer cell interaction with the tumor microenvironment [1]. Many clinical trials have been conducted worldwide with anti-angiogenic drugs. In the case of vascular endothelial growth factor (VEGF), anti-VEGF antibody "bevacizumab" increases overall survival or progression-free survival of patients with metastatic colorectal cancer, non–small cell lung cancer, and breast cancer when given in combination with conventional chemotherapeutic regimens [185].

Targeting Tumor Residence Cells

Many immune infiltrates continue to traffic and reside in the tumor microenvironment such as monocytes, neutrophils, and T cells, Regulatory T cells (Tregs) are also found throughout the body, and contribute to tumor growth. For example, systemic anti-CTLA4 therapy utilizes high expression of CTLA4 on intratumoral Tregs [186 - 188]. However, most common side effects of anti-CTLA4 therapy are colitis and thyroiditis, which may result from loss of Tregs in these tissues [189].

Targeting CAFs

CAFs are able to enhance tumorigenecity, angiogenesis, and metastatic dissemination of cancer cells in comparison to normal fibroblasts [75]. Interestingly, CAFs express a membrane-bound serine protease called fibroblast activation protein α (FAP) that is not detected in normal fibroblasts. However, several phase I and II clinical studies targeting FAP using a humanized monoclonal antibody (sibrotuzumab) failed to produce clinical benefits in colon and non–small cell lung cancer. Based on such data generated by directly targeting FAP at TME, an alternative approach could be using the enzymatic activity of FAP localized specifically in the tumor stroma to activate cytotoxic prodrugs. This strategy is expected to enhance drug efficacy delivered in the TME [190].

Remodeling/Targeting ECM

One of the most important components of ECM that plays a key role in tumor cell adhesion and migration within the TME is hyaluronan (so-called hyaluronic acid (HA) or hyaluronate). HA, modulates the extracellular water and interacts with cellular elements such as receptors. HA plays a crucial role in signaling pathways and cancer biofunctions. HA removal can lead to remodeling of the tumor stroma, development of tumor blood vessels, acceleration of anticancer agent penetration into tumor [191, 192]. Recent studies suggest that administration of exogenous hyaluronidase can impose significant anticancer activity in HA-overexpressing tumors [193]. However local endogenous hyaluronidase expression within the TME can function as a cancer-promoting agent in various solid tumors [194, 195].

Fundamental understanding of TME is mandatory for the development of new therapeutic approaches. Behavior of tumor cells on their own is now known as completely different compared to where they have a microenvironment surrounding them. The development of rational drug combinations that can simultaneously target tumor cells and their microenvironment may represent a solution to overcome therapeutic resistance.

CONSENT FOR PUBLICATION

Not applicable.

CONFLICT OF INTEREST

The authors confirm that the contents of this chapter have no conflict of interest.

ACKNOWLEDGEMENTS

Declared none.

REFERENCES

[1] Hanahan D, Weinberg RA. Hallmarks of cancer: the next generation. Cell 2011; 144(5): 646-74.
[http://dx.doi.org/10.1016/j.cell.2011.02.013] [PMID: 21376230]

[2] Ocaña MC, Martínez-Poveda B, Quesada AR, Medina MÁ. Metabolism within the tumor microenvironment and its implication on cancer progression: An ongoing therapeutic target. Med Res Rev 2019; 39(1): 70-113.
[http://dx.doi.org/10.1002/med.21511] [PMID: 29785785]

[3] Nyberg P, Salo T, Kalluri R. Tumor microenvironment and angiogenesis. Front Biosci 2008; 13: 6537-53.
[http://dx.doi.org/10.2741/3173] [PMID: 18508679]

[4] Fridman WH, Pagès F, Sautès-Fridman C, Galon J. The immune contexture in human tumours: impact on clinical outcome. Nat Rev Cancer 2012; 12(4): 298-306.
[http://dx.doi.org/10.1038/nrc3245] [PMID: 22419253]

[5] Strauss L, Bergmann C, Gooding W, Johnson JT, Whiteside TL. The frequency and suppressor function of CD4+CD25highFoxp3+ T cells in the circulation of patients with squamous cell carcinoma of the head and neck. Clin Cancer Res 2007; 13(21): 6301-11.
[http://dx.doi.org/10.1158/1078-0432.CCR-07-1403] [PMID: 17975141]

[6] Chen L, Wang S, Wang Y, *et al.* IL-6 influences the polarization of macrophages and the formation and growth of colorectal tumor. Oncotarget 2018; 9(25): 17443-54.
[http://dx.doi.org/10.18632/oncotarget.24734] [PMID: 29707119]

[7] Kaimala S, Al-Sbiei A, Cabral-Marques O, Fernandez-Cabezudo MJ, Al-Ramadi BK. Attenuated Bacteria as Immunotherapeutic Tools for Cancer Treatment. Front Oncol 2018; 8: 136.
[http://dx.doi.org/10.3389/fonc.2018.00136] [PMID: 29765907]

[8] Wang JC, Sun X, Ma Q, *et al.* Metformin's antitumour and anti-angiogenic activities are mediated by skewing macrophage polarization. J Cell Mol Med 2018.
[http://dx.doi.org/10.1111/jcmm.13655] [PMID: 29726618]

[9] Tan B, Shi X, Zhang J, *et al.* Inhibition of Rspo-Lgr4 facilitates checkpoint blockade therapy by switching macrophage polarization. Cancer Res 2018; 78(17): 4929-42.
[http://dx.doi.org/10.1158/0008-5472.CAN-18-0152] [PMID: 29967265]

[10] Tan YS, Sansanaphongpricha K, Xie Y, *et al.* Mitigating SOX2-potentiated immune escape of head and neck squamous cell carcinomawith a STING-inducing nanosatellite vaccine. Clin Cancer Res 2018; 24(17): 4242-55.
[http://dx.doi.org/10.1158/1078-0432.CCR-17-2807] [PMID: 29769207]

[11] Baek JH, Yim JH, Song JY, *et al.* Knockdown of end-binding protein 1 induces apoptosis in radioresistant A549 lung cancer cells *via* p38 kinase-dependent COX-2 upregulation. Oncol Rep 2018; 39(4): 1565-72.
[http://dx.doi.org/10.3892/or.2018.6278] [PMID: 29484424]

[12] Hall B, Andreeff M, Marini F. The participation of mesenchymal stem cells in tumor stroma formation and their application as targeted-gene delivery vehicles. Handb Exp Pharmacol 2007; (180): 263-83.
[http://dx.doi.org/10.1007/978-3-540-68976-8_12] [PMID: 17554513]

[13] Guerriero JL. Macrophages: The road less traveled, changing anticancer therapy. Trends Mol Med 2018; 24(5): 472-89.
[http://dx.doi.org/10.1016/j.molmed.2018.03.006] [PMID: 29655673]

[14]   Van Overmeire E, Laoui D, Keirsse J, Van Ginderachter JA, Sarukhan A. Mechanisms driving macrophage diversity and specialization in distinct tumor microenvironments and parallelisms with other tissues. Front Immunol 2014; 5: 127.
[http://dx.doi.org/10.3389/fimmu.2014.00127] [PMID: 24723924]

[15]   Kumar V, Patel S, Tcyganov E, Gabrilovich DI. The nature of myeloid-derived suppressor cells in the tumor microenvironment. Trends Immunol 2016; 37(3): 208-20.
[http://dx.doi.org/10.1016/j.it.2016.01.004] [PMID: 26858199]

[16]   Yin Z, Li C, Wang J, Xue L. Myeloid-derived suppressor cells: Roles in the tumor microenvironment and tumor radiotherapy. Int J Cancer 2019; 144(5): 933-46.
[http://dx.doi.org/10.1002/ijc.31744] [PMID: 29992569]

[17]   Shen M, Wang J, Yu W, *et al.* A novel MDSC-induced PD-1⁻PD-L1⁻ B-cell subset in breast tumor microenvironment possesses immuno-suppressive properties. OncoImmunology 2018; 7(4): e1413520.
[http://dx.doi.org/10.1080/2162402X.2017.1413520] [PMID: 29632731]

[18]   Hurt B, Schulick R, Edil B, El Kasmi KC, Barnett C Jr. Cancer-promoting mechanisms of tumor-associated neutrophils. Am J Surg 2017; 214(5): 938-44.
[http://dx.doi.org/10.1016/j.amjsurg.2017.08.003] [PMID: 28830617]

[19]   Mensurado S, Rei M, Lança T, *et al.* Tumor-associated neutrophils suppress pro-tumoral IL-17+ γδ T cells through induction of oxidative stress. PLoS Biol 2018; 16(5): e2004990.
[http://dx.doi.org/10.1371/journal.pbio.2004990] [PMID: 29750788]

[20]   Hansen M, Andersen MH. The role of dendritic cells in cancer. Semin Immunopathol 2017; 39(3): 307-16.
[http://dx.doi.org/10.1007/s00281-016-0592-y] [PMID: 27638181]

[21]   Guerra DAP, Paiva AE, Sena IFG, *et al.* Targeting glioblastoma-derived pericytes improves chemotherapeutic outcome. Angiogenesis 2018; 21(4): 667-75.
[http://dx.doi.org/10.1007/s10456-018-9621-x] [PMID: 29761249]

[22]   Reina-Campos M, Shelton PM, Diaz-Meco MT, Moscat J. Metabolic reprograming of the tumor microenvironment by p62 and its partners. Biochim Biophys Acta Rev Cancer 2018; 1870(1): 88-95.
[http://dx.doi.org/10.1016/j.bbcan.2018.04.010] [PMID: 29702207]

[23]   Akutagawa T, Aoki S, Yamamoto-Rikitake M, Iwakiri R, Fujimoto K, Toda S. Cancer-adipose tissue interaction and fluid flow synergistically modulate cell kinetics, HER2 expression, and trastuzumab efficacy in gastric cancer. Gastric Cancer 2018; 21(6): 946-55.
[http://dx.doi.org/10.1007/s10120-018-0829-7] [PMID: 29696406]

[24]   Ahirwar DK, Nasser MW, Ouseph MM, *et al.* Fibroblast-derived CXCL12 promotes breast cancer metastasis by facilitating tumor cell intravasation. Oncogene 2018; 37(32): 4428-42.
[http://dx.doi.org/10.1038/s41388-018-0263-7] [PMID: 29720724]

[25]   Liotta LA, Kohn EC. The microenvironment of the tumour-host interface. Nature 2001; 411(6835): 375-9.
[http://dx.doi.org/10.1038/35077241] [PMID: 11357145]

[26]   Zigrino P, Löffek S, Mauch C. Tumor-stroma interactions: their role in the control of tumor cell invasion. Biochimie 2005; 87(3-4): 321-8.
[http://dx.doi.org/10.1016/j.biochi.2004.10.025] [PMID: 15781319]

[27]   Galon J, Costes A, Sanchez-Cabo F, *et al.* Type, density, and location of immune cells within human colorectal tumors predict clinical outcome. Science 2006; 313(5795): 1960-4.
[http://dx.doi.org/10.1126/science.1129139] [PMID: 17008531]

[28]   Nakano O, Sato M, Naito Y, *et al.* Proliferative activity of intratumoral CD8(+) T-lymphocytes as a prognostic factor in human renal cell carcinoma: clinicopathologic demonstration of antitumor immunity. Cancer Res 2001; 61(13): 5132-6.

[PMID: 11431351]

[29] Bromwich EJ, McArdle PA, Canna K, *et al.* The relationship between T-lymphocyte infiltration, stage, tumour grade and survival in patients undergoing curative surgery for renal cell cancer. Br J Cancer 2003; 89(10): 1906-8.
[http://dx.doi.org/10.1038/sj.bjc.6601400] [PMID: 14612901]

[30] Lee N, Zakka LR, Mihm MC Jr, Schatton T. Tumour-infiltrating lymphocytes in melanoma prognosis andcancerimmunotherapy. Pathology 2016; 48(2): 177-87.
[http://dx.doi.org/10.1016/j.pathol.2015.12.006] [PMID: 27020390]

[31] Afkarian M, Sedy JR, Yang J, *et al.* T-bet is a STAT1-induced regulator of IL-12R expression in naïve CD4+ T cells. Nat Immunol 2002; 3(6): 549-57.
[http://dx.doi.org/10.1038/ni794] [PMID: 12006974]

[32] Zhu J, Yamane H, Cote-Sierra J, Guo L, Paul WE. GATA-3 promotes Th2 responses through three different mechanisms: induction of Th2 cytokine production, selective growth of Th2 cells and inhibition of Th1 cell-specific factors. Cell Res 2006; 16(1): 3-10.
[http://dx.doi.org/10.1038/sj.cr.7310002] [PMID: 16467870]

[33] Veldhoen M, Hocking RJ, Atkins CJ, Locksley RM, Stockinger B. TGFbeta in the context of an inflammatory cytokine milieu supports *de novo* differentiation of IL-17-producing T cells. Immunity 2006; 24(2): 179-89.
[http://dx.doi.org/10.1016/j.immuni.2006.01.001] [PMID: 16473830]

[34] Veldhoen M, Uyttenhove C, van Snick J, *et al.* Transforming growth factor-beta 'reprograms' the differentiation of T helper 2 cells and promotes an interleukin 9-producing subset. Nat Immunol 2008; 9(12): 1341-6.
[http://dx.doi.org/10.1038/ni.1659] [PMID: 18931678]

[35] Fazilleau N, Mark L, McHeyzer-Williams LJ, McHeyzer-Williams MG. Follicular helper T cells: lineage and location. Immunity 2009; 30(3): 324-35.
[http://dx.doi.org/10.1016/j.immuni.2009.03.003] [PMID: 19303387]

[36] Luckheeram RV, Zhou R, Verma AD, Xia B. CD4⁻T cells: differentiation and functions. Clin Dev Immunol 2012; 2012: 925135.
[http://dx.doi.org/10.1155/2012/925135] [PMID: 22474485]

[37] Ostroumov D, Fekete-Drimusz N, Saborowski M, Kühnel F, Woller N. CD4 and CD8 T lymphocyte interplay in controlling tumor growth. Cell Mol Life Sci 2018; 75(4): 689-713.
[http://dx.doi.org/10.1007/s00018-017-2686-7] [PMID: 29032503]

[38] Pauken KE, Wherry EJ. Overcoming T cell exhaustion in infection and cancer. Trends Immunol 2015; 36(4): 265-76.
[http://dx.doi.org/10.1016/j.it.2015.02.008] [PMID: 25797516]

[39] Maj T, Wei S, Welling T, Zou W. T cells and costimulation in cancer. Cancer J 2013; 19(6): 473-82.
[http://dx.doi.org/10.1097/PPO.0000000000000002] [PMID: 24270346]

[40] Oleinika K, Nibbs RJ, Graham GJ, Fraser AR. Suppression, subversion and escape: the role of regulatory T cells in cancer progression. Clin Exp Immunol 2013; 171(1): 36-45.
[http://dx.doi.org/10.1111/j.1365-2249.2012.04657.x] [PMID: 23199321]

[41] Qin Z, Richter G, Schüler T, Ibe S, Cao X, Blankenstein T. B cells inhibit induction of T cell-dependent tumor immunity. Nat Med 1998; 4(5): 627-30.
[http://dx.doi.org/10.1038/nm0598-627] [PMID: 9585241]

[42] Inoue S, Leitner WW, Golding B, Scott D. Inhibitory effects of B cells on antitumor immunity. Cancer Res 2006; 66(15): 7741-7.
[http://dx.doi.org/10.1158/0008-5472.CAN-05-3766] [PMID: 16885377]

[43] LeBien TW, Tedder TF. B lymphocytes: how they develop and function. Blood 2008; 112(5): 1570-80.

[http://dx.doi.org/10.1182/blood-2008-02-078071] [PMID: 18725575]

[44]   Schultz GA. Polyadenylic acid-containing of rna in unfertilized and fertilized eggs of the rabbit. Dev Biol 1975; 44(2): 270-7.
[http://dx.doi.org/10.1016/0012-1606(75)90397-8] [PMID: 1169180]

[45]   Milne K, Köbel M, Kalloger SE, *et al.* Systematic analysis of immune infiltrates in high-grade serous ovarian cancer reveals CD20, FoxP3 and TIA-1 as positive prognostic factors. PLoS One 2009; 4(7): e6412.
[http://dx.doi.org/10.1371/journal.pone.0006412] [PMID: 19641607]

[46]   Tsou P, Katayama H, Ostrin EJ, Hanash SM. The emerging role of B cells in tumor immunity. Cancer Res 2016; 76(19): 5597-601.
[http://dx.doi.org/10.1158/0008-5472.CAN-16-0431] [PMID: 27634765]

[47]   Sitrin J, Ring A, Garcia KC, Benoist C, Mathis D. Regulatory T cells control NK cells in an insulitic lesion by depriving them of IL-2. J Exp Med 2013; 210(6): 1153-65.
[http://dx.doi.org/10.1084/jem.20122248] [PMID: 23650440]

[48]   Ghiringhelli F, Ménard C, Terme M, *et al.* CD4+CD25+ regulatory T cells inhibit natural killer cell functions in a transforming growth factor-beta-dependent manner. J Exp Med 2005; 202(8): 1075-85.
[http://dx.doi.org/10.1084/jem.20051511] [PMID: 16230475]

[49]   Pietra G, Manzini C, Rivara S, *et al.* Melanoma cells inhibit natural killer cell function by modulating the expression of activating receptors and cytolytic activity. Cancer Res 2012; 72(6): 1407-15.
[http://dx.doi.org/10.1158/0008-5472.CAN-11-2544] [PMID: 22258454]

[50]   Sevko A, Umansky V. Myeloid-derived suppressor cells interact with tumors in terms of myelopoiesis, tumorigenesis and immunosuppression: thick as thieves. J Cancer 2013; 4(1): 3-11.
[http://dx.doi.org/10.7150/jca.5047] [PMID: 23386900]

[51]   Ortiz ML, Lu L, Ramachandran I, Gabrilovich DI. Myeloid-derived suppressor cells in the development of lung cancer. Cancer Immunol Res 2014; 2(1): 50-8.
[http://dx.doi.org/10.1158/2326-6066.CIR-13-0129] [PMID: 24778162]

[52]   Condamine T, Ramachandran I, Youn JI, Gabrilovich DI. Regulation of tumor metastasis by myeloid-derived suppressor cells. Annu Rev Med 2015; 66: 97-110.
[http://dx.doi.org/10.1146/annurev-med-051013-052304] [PMID: 25341012]

[53]   Casella I, Feccia T, Chelucci C, *et al.* Autocrine-paracrine VEGF loops potentiate the maturation of megakaryocytic precursors through Flt1 receptor. Blood 2003; 101(4): 1316-23.
[http://dx.doi.org/10.1182/blood-2002-07-2184] [PMID: 12406876]

[54]   Tartour E, Pere H, Maillere B, *et al.* Angiogenesis and immunity: a bidirectional link potentially relevant for the monitoring of antiangiogenic therapy and the development of novel therapeutic combination with immunotherapy. Cancer Metastasis Rev 2011; 30(1): 83-95.
[http://dx.doi.org/10.1007/s10555-011-9281-4] [PMID: 21249423]

[55]   Shojaei F, Wu X, Qu X, *et al.* G-CSF-initiated myeloid cell mobilization and angiogenesis mediate tumor refractoriness to anti-VEGF therapy in mouse models. Proc Natl Acad Sci USA 2009; 106(16): 6742-7.
[http://dx.doi.org/10.1073/pnas.0902280106] [PMID: 19346489]

[56]   Zhao X, Rong L, Zhao X, *et al.* TNF signaling drives myeloid-derived suppressor cell accumulation. J Clin Invest 2012; 122(11): 4094-104.
[http://dx.doi.org/10.1172/JCI64115] [PMID: 23064360]

[57]   Kelly PM, Davison RS, Bliss E, McGee JO. Macrophages in human breast disease: a quantitative immunohistochemical study. Br J Cancer 1988; 57(2): 174-7.
[http://dx.doi.org/10.1038/bjc.1988.36] [PMID: 2833921]

[58]   Qian BZ, Pollard JW. Macrophage diversity enhances tumor progression and metastasis. Cell 2010; 141(1): 39-51.

[http://dx.doi.org/10.1016/j.cell.2010.03.014] [PMID: 20371344]

[59] Mantovani A, Allavena P, Sica A, Balkwill F. Cancer-related inflammation. Nature 2008; 454(7203): 436-44.
[http://dx.doi.org/10.1038/nature07205] [PMID: 18650914]

[60] Condeelis J, Pollard JW. Macrophages: obligate partners for tumor cell migration, invasion, and metastasis. Cell 2006; 124(2): 263-6.
[http://dx.doi.org/10.1016/j.cell.2006.01.007] [PMID: 16439202]

[61] Hellstrand K. Melanoma immunotherapy: a battle against radicals? Trends Immunol 2003; 24(5): 232-3.
[http://dx.doi.org/10.1016/S1471-4906(03)00070-X] [PMID: 12738414]

[62] Martinez FO, Sica A, Mantovani A, Locati M. Macrophage activation and polarization. Front Biosci 2008; 13: 453-61.
[http://dx.doi.org/10.2741/2692] [PMID: 17981560]

[63] Nagaraj S, Schrum AG, Cho HI, Celis E, Gabrilovich DI. Mechanism of T cell tolerance induced by myeloid-derived suppressor cells. J Immunol 2010; 184(6): 3106-16.
[http://dx.doi.org/10.4049/jimmunol.0902661] [PMID: 20142361]

[64] Mishalian I, Bayuh R, Levy L, Zolotarov L, Michaeli J, Fridlender ZG. Tumor-associated neutrophils (TAN) develop pro-tumorigenic properties during tumor progression. Cancer Immunol Immunother 2013; 62(11): 1745-56.
[http://dx.doi.org/10.1007/s00262-013-1476-9] [PMID: 24092389]

[65] Engelhardt JJ, Boldajipour B, Beemiller P, *et al.* Marginating dendritic cells of the tumor microenvironment cross-present tumor antigens and stably engage tumor-specific T cells. Cancer Cell 2012; 21(3): 402-17.
[http://dx.doi.org/10.1016/j.ccr.2012.01.008] [PMID: 22439936]

[66] Butt AQ, Mills KH. Immunosuppressive networks and checkpoints controlling antitumor immunity and their blockade in the development of cancer immunotherapeutics and vaccines. Oncogene 2014; 33(38): 4623-31.
[http://dx.doi.org/10.1038/onc.2013.432] [PMID: 24141774]

[67] Tran Janco JM, Lamichhane P, Karyampudi L, Knutson KL. Tumor-infiltrating dendritic cells in cancer pathogenesis. J Immunol 2015; 194(7): 2985-91.
[http://dx.doi.org/10.4049/jimmunol.1403134] [PMID: 25795789]

[68] Nieman KM, Kenny HA, Penicka CV, *et al.* Adipocytes promote ovarian cancer metastasis and provide energy for rapid tumor growth. Nat Med 2011; 17(11): 1498-503.
[http://dx.doi.org/10.1038/nm.2492] [PMID: 22037646]

[69] Donohoe CL, O'Farrell NJ, Doyle SL, Reynolds JV. The role of obesity in gastrointestinal cancer: evidence and opinion. Therap Adv Gastroenterol 2014; 7(1): 38-50.
[http://dx.doi.org/10.1177/1756283X13501786] [PMID: 24381646]

[70] Lago F, Gómez R, Gómez-Reino JJ, Dieguez C, Gualillo O. Adipokines as novel modulators of lipid metabolism. Trends Biochem Sci 2009; 34(10): 500-10.
[http://dx.doi.org/10.1016/j.tibs.2009.06.008] [PMID: 19729309]

[71] Karvonen HM, Lehtonen ST, Sormunen RT, Lappi-Blanco E, Sköld CM, Kaarteenaho RL. Lung cancer-associated myofibroblasts reveal distinctive ultrastructure and function. J Thorac Oncol 2014; 9(5): 664-74.
[http://dx.doi.org/10.1097/JTO.0000000000000149] [PMID: 24662457]

[72] Karki S, Surolia R, Hock TD, *et al.* Wilms' tumor 1 (Wt1) regulates pleural mesothelial cell plasticity and transition into myofibroblasts in idiopathic pulmonary fibrosis. FASEB J 2014; 28(3): 1122-31.
[http://dx.doi.org/10.1096/fj.13-236828] [PMID: 24265486]

[73] Shu H, Li HF. Prognostic effect of stromal myofibroblasts in lung adenocarcinoma. Neoplasma 2012;

59(6): 658-61.
[http://dx.doi.org/10.4149/neo_2012_083] [PMID: 22862165]

[74]   Grotendorst GR, Rahmanie H, Duncan MR. Combinatorial signaling pathways determine fibroblast proliferation and myofibroblast differentiation. FASEB J 2004; 18(3): 469-79.
[http://dx.doi.org/10.1096/fj.03-0699com] [PMID: 15003992]

[75]   Karagiannis GS, Poutahidis T, Erdman SE, Kirsch R, Riddell RH, Diamandis EP. Cancer-associated fibroblasts drive the progression of metastasis through both paracrine and mechanical pressure on cancer tissue. Mol Cancer Res 2012; 10(11): 1403-18.
[http://dx.doi.org/10.1158/1541-7786.MCR-12-0307] [PMID: 23024188]

[76]   Dewald JH, Colomb F, Bobowski-Gerard M, Groux-Degroote S, Delannoy P. Role of cytokine-induced glycosylation changes in regulating cell interactions and cell signaling in inflammatory diseases and cancer. Cells 2016; 5(4): E43.
[http://dx.doi.org/10.3390/cells5040043] [PMID: 27916834]

[77]   Hanahan D, Weinberg RA. The hallmarks of cancer. Cell 2000; 100(1): 57-70.
[http://dx.doi.org/10.1016/S0092-8674(00)81683-9] [PMID: 10647931]

[78]   Thomson AW, Lotze MT. The Cytokine Handbook. Amsterdam, Boston: Academic Press 2003.

[79]   Schwartz DM, Bonelli M, Gadina M, O'Shea JJ. Type I/II cytokines, JAKs, and new strategies for treating autoimmune diseases. Nat Rev Rheumatol 2016; 12(1): 25-36.
[http://dx.doi.org/10.1038/nrrheum.2015.167] [PMID: 26633291]

[80]   Bazan JF. Haemopoietic receptors and helical cytokines. Immunol Today 1990; 11(10): 350-4.
[http://dx.doi.org/10.1016/0167-5699(90)90139-Z] [PMID: 2171545]

[81]   Cosman D. The hematopoietin receptor superfamily. Cytokine 1993; 5(2): 95-106.
[http://dx.doi.org/10.1016/1043-4666(93)90047-9] [PMID: 8392875]

[82]   Haileamlak A. Is public health system in LMICs ready to respond to the ever growing NCDs? Ethiop J Health Sci 2015; 25(3): 198.
[http://dx.doi.org/10.4314/ejhs.v25i3.1] [PMID: 26633921]

[83]   Decker T, Müller M, Stockinger S. The yin and yang of type I interferon activity in bacterial infection. Nat Rev Immunol 2005; 5(9): 675-87.
[http://dx.doi.org/10.1038/nri1684] [PMID: 16110316]

[84]   Hervas-Stubbs S, Perez-Gracia JL, Rouzaut A, Sanmamed MF, Le Bon A, Melero I. Direct effects of type I interferons on cells of the immune system. Clin Cancer Res 2011; 17(9): 2619-27.
[http://dx.doi.org/10.1158/1078-0432.CCR-10-1114] [PMID: 21372217]

[85]   Pestka S, Krause CD, Walter MR. Interferons, interferon-like cytokines, and their receptors. Immunol Rev 2004; 202: 8-32.
[http://dx.doi.org/10.1111/j.0105-2896.2004.00204.x] [PMID: 15546383]

[86]   Capobianchi MR, Uleri E, Caglioti C, Dolei A. Type I IFN family members: similarity, differences and interaction. Cytokine Growth Factor Rev 2015; 26(2): 103-11.
[http://dx.doi.org/10.1016/j.cytogfr.2014.10.011] [PMID: 25466633]

[87]   Wheelock EF. Interferon-Like Virus-Inhibitor Induced in Human Leukocytes by Phytohemagglutinin. Science 1965; 149(3681): 310-1.
[http://dx.doi.org/10.1126/science.149.3681.310]

[88]   Gray PW, Goeddel DV. Structure of the human immune interferon gene. Nature 1982; 298(5877): 859-63.
[http://dx.doi.org/10.1038/298859a0] [PMID: 6180322]

[89]   Sheppard P, Kindsvogel W, Xu W, *et al.* IL-28, IL-29 and their class II cytokine receptor IL-28R. Nat Immunol 2003; 4(1): 63-8.
[http://dx.doi.org/10.1038/ni873] [PMID: 12469119]

[90]   Iversen MB, Paludan SR. Mechanisms of type III interferon expression. J Interferon Cytokine Res 2010; 30(8): 573-8.
[http://dx.doi.org/10.1089/jir.2010.0063] [PMID: 20645874]

[91]   Hedrich CM, Bream JH. Cell type-specific regulation of IL-10 expression in inflammation and disease. Immunol Res 2010; 47(1-3): 185-206.
[http://dx.doi.org/10.1007/s12026-009-8150-5] [PMID: 20087682]

[92]   Jankovic D, Kugler DG, Sher A. IL-10 production by CD4+ effector T cells: a mechanism for self-regulation. Mucosal Immunol 2010; 3(3): 239-46.
[http://dx.doi.org/10.1038/mi.2010.8] [PMID: 20200511]

[93]   Jankovic D, Kullberg MC, Feng CG, *et al.* Conventional T-bet(+)Foxp3(-) Th1 cells are the major source of host-protective regulatory IL-10 during intracellular protozoan infection. J Exp Med 2007; 204(2): 273-83.
[http://dx.doi.org/10.1084/jem.20062175] [PMID: 17283209]

[94]   Maynard CL, Weaver CT. Diversity in the contribution of interleukin-10 to T-cell-mediated immune regulation. Immunol Rev 2008; 226: 219-33.
[http://dx.doi.org/10.1111/j.1600-065X.2008.00711.x] [PMID: 19161427]

[95]   McGeachy MJ, Bak-Jensen KS, Chen Y, *et al.* TGF-beta and IL-6 drive the production of IL-17 and IL-10 by T cells and restrain T(H)-17 cell-mediated pathology. Nat Immunol 2007; 8(12): 1390-7.
[http://dx.doi.org/10.1038/ni1539] [PMID: 17994024]

[96]   Mocellin S, Marincola F, Rossi CR, Nitti D, Lise M. The multifaceted relationship between IL-10 and adaptive immunity: putting together the pieces of a puzzle. Cytokine Growth Factor Rev 2004; 15(1): 61-76.
[http://dx.doi.org/10.1016/j.cytogfr.2003.11.001] [PMID: 14746814]

[97]   Umetsu SE, Winandy S. Ikaros is a regulator of Il10 expression in CD4+ T cells. J Immunol 2009; 183(9): 5518-25.
[http://dx.doi.org/10.4049/jimmunol.0901284] [PMID: 19828627]

[98]   Chu CQ. How much have we learnt about the TNF family of cytokines? Cytokine 2018; 101: 1-3.
[http://dx.doi.org/10.1016/j.cyto.2017.05.004] [PMID: 28527660]

[99]   Dinarello CA. Immunological and inflammatory functions of the interleukin-1 family. Annu Rev Immunol 2009; 27: 519-50.
[http://dx.doi.org/10.1146/annurev.immunol.021908.132612] [PMID: 19302047]

[100] Garlanda C, Dinarello CA, Mantovani A. The interleukin-1 family: back to the future. Immunity 2013; 39(6): 1003-18.
[http://dx.doi.org/10.1016/j.immuni.2013.11.010] [PMID: 24332029]

[101] Bassoy EY, Towne JE, Gabay C. Regulation and function of interleukin-36 cytokines. Immunol Rev 2018; 281(1): 169-78.
[http://dx.doi.org/10.1111/imr.12610] [PMID: 29247994]

[102] Dinarello CA. The IL-1 family and inflammatory diseases. Clin Exp Rheumatol 2002; 20(5) (Suppl. 27): S1-S13.
[PMID: 14989423]

[103] Aggarwal S, Gurney AL. IL-17: prototype member of an emerging cytokine family. J Leukoc Biol 2002; 71(1): 1-8.
[PMID: 11781375]

[104] Toy D, Kugler D, Wolfson M, *et al.* Cutting edge: interleukin 17 signals through a heteromeric receptor complex. J Immunol 2006; 177(1): 36-9.
[http://dx.doi.org/10.4049/jimmunol.177.1.36] [PMID: 16785495]

[105] Rickel EA, Siegel LA, Yoon BR, *et al.* Identification of functional roles for both IL-17RB and IL-

17RA in mediating IL-25-induced activities. J Immunol 2008; 181(6): 4299-310.
[http://dx.doi.org/10.4049/jimmunol.181.6.4299] [PMID: 18768888]

[106] Ramirez-Carrozzi V, Sambandam A, Luis E, *et al.* IL-17C regulates the innate immune function of epithelial cells in an autocrine manner. Nat Immunol 2011; 12(12): 1159-66.
[http://dx.doi.org/10.1038/ni.2156] [PMID: 21993848]

[107] Moser B, Wolf M, Walz A, Loetscher P. Chemokines: multiple levels of leukocyte migration control. Trends Immunol 2004; 25(2): 75-84.
[http://dx.doi.org/10.1016/j.it.2003.12.005] [PMID: 15102366]

[108] Charo IF, Ransohoff RM. The many roles of chemokines and chemokine receptors in inflammation. N Engl J Med 2006; 354(6): 610-21.
[http://dx.doi.org/10.1056/NEJMra052723] [PMID: 16467548]

[109] Huma ZE, Sanchez J, Lim HD, *et al.* Key determinants of selective binding and activation by the monocyte chemoattractant proteins at the chemokine receptor CCR2. Sci Signal 2017; 10(480): eaai8529.
[http://dx.doi.org/10.1126/scisignal.aai8529] [PMID: 28536301]

[110] Rot A, von Andrian UH. Chemokines in innate and adaptive host defense: basic chemokinese grammar for immune cells. Annu Rev Immunol 2004; 22: 891-928.
[http://dx.doi.org/10.1146/annurev.immunol.22.012703.104543] [PMID: 15032599]

[111] Griffith JW, Sokol CL, Luster AD. Chemokines and chemokine receptors: positioning cells for host defense and immunity. Annu Rev Immunol 2014; 32: 659-702.
[http://dx.doi.org/10.1146/annurev-immunol-032713-120145] [PMID: 24655300]

[112] Atretkhany KN, Drutskaya MS, Nedospasov SA, Grivennikov SI, Kuprash DV. Chemokines, cytokines and exosomes help tumors to shape inflammatory microenvironment. Pharmacol Ther 2016; 168: 98-112.
[http://dx.doi.org/10.1016/j.pharmthera.2016.09.011] [PMID: 27613100]

[113] Sporn MB, Todaro GJ. Autocrine secretion and malignant transformation of cells. N Engl J Med 1980; 303(15): 878-80.
[http://dx.doi.org/10.1056/NEJM198010093031511] [PMID: 7412807]

[114] Witsch E, Sela M, Yarden Y. Roles for growth factors in cancer progression. Physiology (Bethesda) 2010; 25(2): 85-101.
[http://dx.doi.org/10.1152/physiol.00045.2009] [PMID: 20430953]

[115] Youness RA, Rahmoon MA, Assal RA, *et al.* Contradicting interplay between insulin-like growth factor-1 and miR-486-5p in primary NK cells and hepatoma cell lines with a contemporary inhibitory impact on HCC tumor progression. Growth Factors 2016; 34(3-4): 128-40.
[http://dx.doi.org/10.1080/08977194.2016.1200571] [PMID: 27388576]

[116] Suhovskih AV, Mostovich LA, Kunin IS, *et al.* Proteoglycan expression in normal human prostate tissue and prostate cancer. ISRN Oncol 2013; 2013: 680136.
[http://dx.doi.org/10.1155/2013/680136] [PMID: 23691363]

[117] Blehm BH, Jiang N, Kotobuki Y, Tanner K. Deconstructing the role of the ECM microenvironment on drug efficacy targeting MAPK signaling in a pre-clinical platform for cutaneous melanoma. Biomaterials 2015; 56: 129-39.
[http://dx.doi.org/10.1016/j.biomaterials.2015.03.041] [PMID: 25934286]

[118] Fullár A, Dudás J, Oláh L, *et al.* Remodeling of extracellular matrix by normal and tumor-associated fibroblasts promotes cervical cancer progression. BMC Cancer 2015; 15: 256.
[http://dx.doi.org/10.1186/s12885-015-1272-3] [PMID: 25885552]

[119] de Kruijf EM, van Nes JG, van de Velde CJ, *et al.* Tumor-stroma ratio in the primary tumor is a prognostic factor in early breast cancer patients, especially in triple-negative carcinoma patients. Breast Cancer Res Treat 2011; 125(3): 687-96.

[http://dx.doi.org/10.1007/s10549-010-0855-6] [PMID: 20361254]

[120] Suhovskih AV, Aidagulova SV, Kashuba VI, Grigorieva EV. Proteoglycans as potential microenvironmental biomarkers for colon cancer. Cell Tissue Res 2015; 361(3): 833-44.
[http://dx.doi.org/10.1007/s00441-015-2141-8] [PMID: 25715761]

[121] Januchowski R, Zawierucha P, Ruciński M, Nowicki M, Zabel M. Extracellular matrix proteins expression profiling in chemoresistant variants of the A2780 ovarian cancer cell line. BioMed Res Int 2014; 2014: 365867.
[http://dx.doi.org/10.1155/2014/365867] [PMID: 24804215]

[122] Lamouille S, Xu J, Derynck R. Molecular mechanisms of epithelial-mesenchymal transition. Nat Rev Mol Cell Biol 2014; 15(3): 178-96.
[http://dx.doi.org/10.1038/nrm3758] [PMID: 24556840]

[123] Cataisson C, Salcedo R, Hakim S, *et al.* IL-1R-MyD88 signaling in keratinocyte transformation and carcinogenesis. J Exp Med 2012; 209(9): 1689-702.
[http://dx.doi.org/10.1084/jem.20101355] [PMID: 22908325]

[124] Borrelli C, Ricci B, Vulpis E, *et al.* Drug-induced senescent multiple myeloma cells elicit NK cell proliferation by direct or exosome-mediated IL15 *Trans*-presentation. Cancer Immunol Res 2018; 6(7): 860-9.
[http://dx.doi.org/10.1158/2326-6066.CIR-17-0604] [PMID: 29691234]

[125] Locati M, Mantovani A, Sica A. Macrophage activation and polarization as an adaptive component of innate immunity. Adv Immunol 2013; 120: 163-84.
[http://dx.doi.org/10.1016/B978-0-12-417028-5.00006-5] [PMID: 24070384]

[126] Allavena P, Mantovani A. Immunology in the clinic review series; focus on cancer: tumour-associated macrophages: undisputed stars of the inflammatory tumour microenvironment. Clin Exp Immunol 2012; 167(2): 195-205.
[http://dx.doi.org/10.1111/j.1365-2249.2011.04515.x] [PMID: 22235995]

[127] Ostrand-Rosenberg S, Sinha P. Myeloid-derived suppressor cells: linking inflammation and cancer. J Immunol 2009; 182(8): 4499-506.
[http://dx.doi.org/10.4049/jimmunol.0802740] [PMID: 19342621]

[128] Gaggianesi M, Turdo A, Chinnici A, *et al.* IL4 primes the dynamics of breast cancer progression *via* DUSP4 inhibition. Cancer Res 2017; 77(12): 3268-79.
[http://dx.doi.org/10.1158/0008-5472.CAN-16-3126] [PMID: 28400477]

[129] Li P, Shan JX, Chen XH, *et al.* Epigenetic silencing of microRNA-149 in cancer-associated fibroblasts mediates prostaglandin E2/interleukin-6 signaling in the tumor microenvironment. Cell Res 2015; 25(5): 588-603.
[http://dx.doi.org/10.1038/cr.2015.51] [PMID: 25916550]

[130] Ohno Y, Kitamura H, Takahashi N, *et al.* IL-6 down-regulates HLA class II expression and IL-12 production of human dendritic cells to impair activation of antigen-specific CD4(+) T cells. Cancer Immunol Immunother 2016; 65(2): 193-204.
[http://dx.doi.org/10.1007/s00262-015-1791-4] [PMID: 26759006]

[131] Kumari N, Dwarakanath BS, Das A, Bhatt AN. Role of interleukin-6 in cancer progression and therapeutic resistance. Tumour Biol 2016; 37(9): 11553-72.
[http://dx.doi.org/10.1007/s13277-016-5098-7] [PMID: 27260630]

[132] Ortiz-Montero P, Londoño-Vallejo A, Vernot JP. Senescence-associated IL-6 and IL-8 cytokines induce a self- and cross-reinforced senescence/inflammatory milieu strengthening tumorigenic capabilities in the MCF-7 breast cancer cell line. Cell Commun Signal 2017; 15(1): 17.
[http://dx.doi.org/10.1186/s12964-017-0172-3] [PMID: 28472950]

[133] Sato T, Terai M, Tamura Y, Alexeev V, Mastrangelo MJ, Selvan SR. Interleukin 10 in the tumor microenvironment: a target for anticancer immunotherapy. Immunol Res 2011; 51(2-3): 170-82.

[http://dx.doi.org/10.1007/s12026-011-8262-6] [PMID: 22139852]

[134] García-Hernández ML, Hernández-Pando R, Gariglio P, Berumen J. Interleukin-10 promotes B16-melanoma growth by inhibition of macrophage functions and induction of tumour and vascular cell proliferation. Immunology 2002; 105(2): 231-43.
[http://dx.doi.org/10.1046/j.1365-2567.2002.01363.x] [PMID: 11872099]

[135] Berti FCB, Pereira APL, Cebinelli GCM, Trugilo KP, Brajão de Oliveira K. The role of interleukin 10 in human papilloma virus infection and progression to cervical carcinoma. Cytokine Growth Factor Rev 2017; 34: 1-13.
[http://dx.doi.org/10.1016/j.cytogfr.2017.03.002] [PMID: 28365229]

[136] Berraondo P, Etxeberria I, Ponz-Sarvise M, Melero I. Revisiting Interleukin-12 as a Cancer Immunotherapy Agent. Clin Cancer Res 2018; 24(12): 2716-8.
[http://dx.doi.org/10.1158/1078-0432.CCR-18-0381] [PMID: 29549160]

[137] Fujisawa T, Joshi B, Nakajima A, Puri RK. A novel role of interleukin-13 receptor alpha2 in pancreatic cancer invasion and metastasis. Cancer Res 2009; 69(22): 8678-85.
[http://dx.doi.org/10.1158/0008-5472.CAN-09-2100] [PMID: 19887609]

[138] Barderas R, Bartolomé RA, Fernandez-Aceñero MJ, Torres S, Casal JI. High expression of IL-13 receptor α2 in colorectal cancer is associated with invasion, liver metastasis, and poor prognosis. Cancer Res 2012; 72(11): 2780-90.
[http://dx.doi.org/10.1158/0008-5472.CAN-11-4090] [PMID: 22505647]

[139] Mlecnik B, Bindea G, Angell HK, *et al.* Functional network pipeline reveals genetic determinants associated with *in situ* lymphocyte proliferation and survival of cancer patients. Sci Transl Med 2014; 6(228): 228ra37.
[http://dx.doi.org/10.1126/scitranslmed.3007240] [PMID: 24648340]

[140] Liu RB, Engels B, Schreiber K, *et al.* IL-15 in tumor microenvironment causes rejection of large established tumors by T cells in a noncognate T cell receptor-dependent manner. Proc Natl Acad Sci USA 2013; 110(20): 8158-63.
[http://dx.doi.org/10.1073/pnas.1301022110] [PMID: 23637340]

[141] Mortier E, Advincula R, Kim L, *et al.* Macrophage- and dendritic-cell-derived interleukin-15 receptor alpha supports homeostasis of distinct CD8+ T cell subsets. Immunity 2009; 31(5): 811-22.
[http://dx.doi.org/10.1016/j.immuni.2009.09.017] [PMID: 19913445]

[142] Anthony SM, Rivas SC, Colpitts SL, Howard ME, Stonier SW, Schluns KS. Inflammatory signals regulate IL-15 in response to lymphodepletion. J Immunol 2016; 196(11): 4544-52.
[http://dx.doi.org/10.4049/jimmunol.1600219] [PMID: 27183627]

[143] Jungnickel C, Schmidt LH, Bittigkoffer L, *et al.* IL-17C mediates the recruitment of tumor-associated neutrophils and lung tumor growth. Oncogene 2017; 36(29): 4182-90.
[http://dx.doi.org/10.1038/onc.2017.28] [PMID: 28346430]

[144] Alipoor SD, Mortaz E, Varahram M, *et al.* The potential biomarkers and immunological effects of tumor-derived exosomes in lung cancer. Front Immunol 2018; 9: 819.
[http://dx.doi.org/10.3389/fimmu.2018.00819] [PMID: 29720982]

[145] Tanaka Y, Nishikawa M, Mizukami Y, *et al.* Control of polarization and tumoricidal activity of macrophages by multicellular spheroid formation. J Control Release 2018; 270: 177-83.
[http://dx.doi.org/10.1016/j.jconrel.2017.12.006] [PMID: 29225184]

[146] Wei L, Eric N, Napoleone F. Interleukin-22 promotes tumor angiogenesis. Angiogenesis 2019; 22(2): 311-23.

[147] Nie W, Yu T, Sang Y, Gao X. Tumor-promoting effect of IL-23 in mammary cancer mediated by infiltration of M2 macrophages and neutrophils in tumor microenvironment. Biochem Biophys Res Commun 2017; 482(4): 1400-6.
[http://dx.doi.org/10.1016/j.bbrc.2016.12.048] [PMID: 27956175]

[148] Miller AM. Role of IL-33 in inflammation and disease. J Inflamm (Lond) 2011; 8(1): 22.
[http://dx.doi.org/10.1186/1476-9255-8-22] [PMID: 21871091]

[149] Pollheimer J, Bodin J, Sundnes O, *et al.* Interleukin-33 drives a proinflammatory endothelial activation that selectively targets nonquiescent cells. Arterioscler Thromb Vasc Biol 2013; 33(2): e47-55.
[http://dx.doi.org/10.1161/ATVBAHA.112.253427] [PMID: 23162017]

[150] Choi YS, Choi HJ, Min JK, *et al.* Interleukin-33 induces angiogenesis and vascular permeability through ST2/TRAF6-mediated endothelial nitric oxide production. Blood 2009; 114(14): 3117-26.
[http://dx.doi.org/10.1182/blood-2009-02-203372] [PMID: 19661270]

[151] Lu B, Yang M, Wang Q. Interleukin-33 in tumorigenesis, tumor immune evasion, and cancer immunotherapy. J Mol Med (Berl) 2016; 94(5): 535-43.
[http://dx.doi.org/10.1007/s00109-016-1397-0] [PMID: 26922618]

[152] Zou JM, Qin J, Li YC, *et al.* IL-35 induces N2 phenotype of neutrophils to promote tumor growth. Oncotarget 2017; 8(20): 33501-14.
[http://dx.doi.org/10.18632/oncotarget.16819] [PMID: 28432279]

[153] Ou W, Thapa RK, Jiang L, *et al.* Regulatory T cell-targeted hybrid nanoparticles combined with immuno-checkpoint blockage for cancer immunotherapy. J Control Release 2018; 281: 84-96.
[http://dx.doi.org/10.1016/j.jconrel.2018.05.018] [PMID: 29777794]

[154] Chen A, Sceneay J, Gödde N, *et al.* Intermittent hypoxia induces a metastatic phenotype in breast cancer. Oncogene 2018; 37(31): 4214-25.
[http://dx.doi.org/10.1038/s41388-018-0259-3] [PMID: 29713057]

[155] Albini A, Bruno A, Noonan DM, Mortara L. Contribution to tumor angiogenesis from innate immune cells within the tumor microenvironment: implications for immunotherapy. Front Immunol 2018; 9: 527.
[http://dx.doi.org/10.3389/fimmu.2018.00527] [PMID: 29675018]

[156] Gangaplara A, Martens C, Dahlstrom E, *et al.* Type I interferon signaling attenuates regulatory T cell function in viral infection and in the tumor microenvironment. PLoS Pathog 2018; 14(4): e1006985.
[http://dx.doi.org/10.1371/journal.ppat.1006985] [PMID: 29672594]

[157] Kryczek I, Lange A, Mottram P, *et al.* CXCL12 and vascular endothelial growth factor synergistically induce neoangiogenesis in human ovarian cancers. Cancer Res 2005; 65(2): 465-72.
[PMID: 15695388]

[158] Zou W, Machelon V, Coulomb-L'Hermin A, *et al.* Stromal-derived factor-1 in human tumors recruits and alters the function of plasmacytoid precursor dendritic cells. Nat Med 2001; 7(12): 1339-46.
[http://dx.doi.org/10.1038/nm1201-1339] [PMID: 11726975]

[159] Bell D, Chomarat P, Broyles D, *et al.* In breast carcinoma tissue, immature dendritic cells reside within the tumor, whereas mature dendritic cells are located in peritumoral areas. J Exp Med 1999; 190(10): 1417-26.
[http://dx.doi.org/10.1084/jem.190.10.1417] [PMID: 10562317]

[160] Kryczek I, Lin Y, Nagarsheth N, *et al.* IL-22(+)CD4(+) T cells promote colorectal cancer stemness *via* STAT3 transcription factor activation and induction of the methyltransferase DOT1L. Immunity 2014; 40(5): 772-84.
[http://dx.doi.org/10.1016/j.immuni.2014.03.010] [PMID: 24816405]

[161] Huang YH, Cao YF, Jiang ZY, Zhang S, Gao F. Th22 cell accumulation is associated with colorectal cancer development. World J Gastroenterol 2015; 21(14): 4216-24.
[http://dx.doi.org/10.3748/wjg.v21.i14.4216] [PMID: 25892871]

[162] Zhuang Y, Peng LS, Zhao YL, *et al.* Increased intratumoral IL-22-producing CD4(+) T cells and Th22 cells correlate with gastric cancer progression and predict poor patient survival. Cancer Immunol Immunother 2012; 61(11): 1965-75.
[http://dx.doi.org/10.1007/s00262-012-1241-5] [PMID: 22527243]

[163] Kuang DM, Xiao X, Zhao Q, *et al.* B7-H1-expressing antigen-presenting cells mediate polarization of protumorigenic Th22 subsets. J Clin Invest 2014; 124(10): 4657-67.
[http://dx.doi.org/10.1172/JCI74381] [PMID: 25244097]

[164] Curiel TJ, Coukos G, Zou L, *et al.* Specific recruitment of regulatory T cells in ovarian carcinoma fosters immune privilege and predicts reduced survival. Nat Med 2004; 10(9): 942-9.
[http://dx.doi.org/10.1038/nm1093] [PMID: 15322536]

[165] Kim CH, Johnston B, Butcher EC. Trafficking machinery of NKT cells: shared and differential chemokine receptor expression among V alpha 24(+)V beta 11(+) NKT cell subsets with distinct cytokine-producing capacity. Blood 2002; 100(1): 11-6.
[http://dx.doi.org/10.1182/blood-2001-12-0196] [PMID: 12070001]

[166] Metelitsa LS, Wu HW, Wang H, *et al.* Natural killer T cells infiltrate neuroblastomas expressing the chemokine CCL2. J Exp Med 2004; 199(9): 1213-21.
[http://dx.doi.org/10.1084/jem.20031462] [PMID: 15123743]

[167] Song L, Ara T, Wu HW, *et al.* Oncogene MYCN regulates localization of NKT cells to the site of disease in neuroblastoma. J Clin Invest 2007; 117(9): 2702-12.
[http://dx.doi.org/10.1172/JCI30751] [PMID: 17710228]

[168] Schmidt M, Böhm D, von Törne C, *et al.* The humoral immune system has a key prognostic impact in node-negative breast cancer. Cancer Res 2008; 68(13): 5405-13.
[http://dx.doi.org/10.1158/0008-5472.CAN-07-5206] [PMID: 18593943]

[169] Kotowicz B, Fuksiewicz M, Jonska-Gmyrek J, *et al.* Clinical significance of pretreatment serum levels of VEGF and its receptors, IL- 8, and their prognostic value in type I and II endometrial cancer patients. PLoS One 2017; 12(10): e0184576.
[http://dx.doi.org/10.1371/journal.pone.0184576] [PMID: 28991928]

[170] Skirnisdottir I, Seidal T, Åkerud H. The relationship of the angiogenesis regulators VEGF-A, VEGF-R1 and VEGF-R2 to p53 status and prognostic factors in epithelial ovarian carcinoma in FIGO-stages I-II. Int J Oncol 2016; 48(3): 998-1006.
[http://dx.doi.org/10.3892/ijo.2016.3333] [PMID: 26783205]

[171] Yu CF, Chen FH, Lu MH, Hong JH, Chiang CS. Dual roles of tumour cells-derived matrix metalloproteinase 2 on brain tumour growth and invasion. Br J Cancer 2017; 117(12): 1828-36.
[http://dx.doi.org/10.1038/bjc.2017.362] [PMID: 29065106]

[172] Vihinen P, Kähäri VM. Matrix metalloproteinases in cancer: prognostic markers and therapeutic targets. Int J Cancer 2002; 99(2): 157-66.
[http://dx.doi.org/10.1002/ijc.10329] [PMID: 11979428]

[173] Illman SA, Lehti K, Keski-Oja J, Lohi J. Epilysin (MMP-28) induces TGF-beta mediated epithelial to mesenchymal transition in lung carcinoma cells. J Cell Sci 2006; 119(Pt 18): 3856-65.
[http://dx.doi.org/10.1242/jcs.03157] [PMID: 16940349]

[174] Thiery JP. Epithelial-mesenchymal transitions in tumour progression. Nat Rev Cancer 2002; 2(6): 442-54.
[http://dx.doi.org/10.1038/nrc822] [PMID: 12189386]

[175] Hanahan D, Coussens LM. Accessories to the crime: functions of cells recruited to the tumor microenvironment. Cancer Cell 2012; 21(3): 309-22.
[http://dx.doi.org/10.1016/j.ccr.2012.02.022] [PMID: 22439926]

[176] Dunn GP, Bruce AT, Ikeda H, Old LJ, Schreiber RD. Cancer immunoediting: from immunosurveillance to tumor escape. Nat Immunol 2002; 3(11): 991-8.
[http://dx.doi.org/10.1038/ni1102-991] [PMID: 12407406]

[177] Vaupel P, Mayer A. Hypoxia in tumors: pathogenesis-related classification, characterization of hypoxia subtypes, and associated biological and clinical implications. Adv Exp Med Biol 2014; 812: 19-24.

[http://dx.doi.org/10.1007/978-1-4939-0620-8_3] [PMID: 24729210]

[178] Vaupel P, Mayer A. Hypoxia in cancer: significance and impact on clinical outcome. Cancer Metastasis Rev 2007; 26(2): 225-39.
[http://dx.doi.org/10.1007/s10555-007-9055-1] [PMID: 17440684]

[179] Sormendi S, Wielockx B. Hypoxia pathway proteins as central mediators of metabolism in the tumor cells and their microenvironment. Front Immunol 2018; 9: 40.
[http://dx.doi.org/10.3389/fimmu.2018.00040] [PMID: 29434587]

[180] Masoud GN, Li W. HIF-1α pathway: role, regulation and intervention for cancer therapy. Acta Pharm Sin B 2015; 5(5): 378-89.
[http://dx.doi.org/10.1016/j.apsb.2015.05.007] [PMID: 26579469]

[181] Ziello JE, Jovin IS, Huang Y. Hypoxia-Inducible Factor (HIF)-1 regulatory pathway and its potential for therapeutic intervention in malignancy and ischemia. Yale J Biol Med 2007; 80(2): 51-60.
[PMID: 18160990]

[182] Yu T, Tang B, Sun X. Development of inhibitors targeting hypoxia-inducible factor 1 and 2 for cancer therapy. Yonsei Med J 2017; 58(3): 489-96.
[http://dx.doi.org/10.3349/ymj.2017.58.3.489] [PMID: 28332352]

[183] Paolicchi E, Gemignani F, Krstic-Demonacos M, Dedhar S, Mutti L, Landi S. Targeting hypoxic response for cancer therapy. Oncotarget 2016; 7(12): 13464-78.
[http://dx.doi.org/10.18632/oncotarget.7229] [PMID: 26859576]

[184] Kang JH, Song KH, Jeong KC, *et al.* Involvement of Cox-2 in the metastatic potential of chemotherapy-resistant breast cancer cells. BMC Cancer 2011; 11: 334.
[http://dx.doi.org/10.1186/1471-2407-11-334] [PMID: 21813027]

[185] Montero AJ, Escobar M, Lopes G, Glück S, Vogel C. Bevacizumab in the treatment of metastatic breast cancer: friend or foe? Curr Oncol Rep 2012; 14(1): 1-11.
[http://dx.doi.org/10.1007/s11912-011-0202-z] [PMID: 22012632]

[186] Bulliard Y, Jolicoeur R, Windman M, *et al.* Activating Fc γ receptors contribute to the antitumor activities of immunoregulatory receptor-targeting antibodies. J Exp Med 2013; 210(9): 1685-93.
[http://dx.doi.org/10.1084/jem.20130573] [PMID: 23897982]

[187] Selby MJ, Engelhardt JJ, Quigley M, *et al.* Anti-CTLA-4 antibodies of IgG2a isotype enhance antitumor activity through reduction of intratumoral regulatory T cells. Cancer Immunol Res 2013; 1(1): 32-42.
[http://dx.doi.org/10.1158/2326-6066.CIR-13-0013] [PMID: 24777248]

[188] Simpson TR, Li F, Montalvo-Ortiz W, *et al.* Fc-dependent depletion of tumor-infiltrating regulatory T cells co-defines the efficacy of anti-CTLA-4 therapy against melanoma. J Exp Med 2013; 210(9): 1695-710.
[http://dx.doi.org/10.1084/jem.20130579] [PMID: 23897981]

[189] Bertrand A, Kostine M, Barnetche T, Truchetet ME, Schaeverbeke T. Immune related adverse events associated with anti-CTLA-4 antibodies: systematic review and meta-analysis. BMC Med 2015; 13: 211.
[http://dx.doi.org/10.1186/s12916-015-0455-8] [PMID: 26337719]

[190] Brennen WN, Rosen DM, Wang H, Isaacs JT, Denmeade SR. Targeting carcinoma-associated fibroblasts within the tumor stroma with a fibroblast activation protein-activated prodrug. J Natl Cancer Inst 2012; 104(17): 1320-34.
[http://dx.doi.org/10.1093/jnci/djs336] [PMID: 22911669]

[191] Toole BP, Hascall VC. Hyaluronan and tumor growth. Am J Pathol 2002; 161(3): 745-7.
[http://dx.doi.org/10.1016/S0002-9440(10)64232-0] [PMID: 12213700]

[192] Kultti A, Li X, Jiang P, Thompson CB, Frost GI, Shepard HM. Therapeutic targeting of hyaluronan in the tumor stroma. Cancers (Basel) 2012; 4(3): 873-903.

[http://dx.doi.org/10.3390/cancers4030873] [PMID: 24213471]

[193]   Brekken C, de Lange Davies C. Hyaluronidase reduces the interstitial fluid pressure in solid tumours in a non-linear concentration-dependent manner. Cancer Lett 1998; 131(1): 65-70.
[http://dx.doi.org/10.1016/S0304-3835(98)00202-X] [PMID: 9839621]

[194]   Lokeshwar VB, Lokeshwar BL, Pham HT, Block NL. Association of elevated levels of hyaluronidase, a matrix-degrading enzyme, with prostate cancer progression. Cancer Res 1996; 56(3): 651-7.
[PMID: 8564986]

[195]   Pham HT, Block NL, Lokeshwar VB. Tumor-derived hyaluronidase: a diagnostic urine marker for high-grade bladder cancer. Cancer Res 1997; 57(4): 778-83.
[PMID: 9044860]

CHAPTER 3

Nanotechnology in Cancer Theranostics

Asmaa Mostafa[1,2] and **Matthias Bartneck**[1,*]

[1] *Department of Internal Medicine III, University Hospital RWTH Aachen, Pauwelsstraße 30, 52074, Aachen, Germany*

[2] *Department of Microbial Biotechnology, Division of Genetic Engineering and Biotechnology, National Research Center, 33 El-Bohouth St., El-Dokki, 12622, Giza, Egypt*

Abstract: Our immune system protects our body from a large number of threats. External threats include pathogens from various sources. Internally, the cells of our immune system continuously fight cancer cells and thereby prevent tumor development. Immunotherapies which employ monoclonal antibodies have significantly enriched our vision of cancer treatment. Unleashing the checkpoint blockade of tumors mobilizes the cytotoxic T cells to eliminate cancer cells, and therefore, amplifies the anti-tumor response of the immune system. The lymphoid immune cells, particularly cytotoxic CD8 T cells, are the current focus of novel interventions such as chimeric antigen receptor (CAR) engineered T cells. Nanomedicines are predestined to target macrophages due to their high phagocytic activity and their large numbers in different types of tumors. Specifically, nanomedical formulations might additionally explore the potential of modulating macrophages as key effector cell which can influence the tumor microenvironment. The therapeutic cargo to be delivered to cells or tissues can benefit from the "Omics" sciences and use knowledge to specifically modulate gene expression and protein generation using small non-coding RNA. Strategies to localize drug delivery have the potential to enrich nanomedicines for their potential ability to be concentrated in certain parts of the body. Such applications can rely, for instance, on magnetic fields or infrared light sensitive systems, in order to increase target specificity. Here, we put an emphasis on the applicability of the strategies to improve target specific accumulation of theranostics and discuss potential improvements of cancer immunotherapies.

Keywords: Cancer immunotherapy, Drug delivery, Imaging, Nanomedicine, Theranostic.

* **Corresponding author Matthias Bartneck:** Department of Medicine III University Hospital Aachen 52074 Aachen, Germany; Tel: -49-241-80662; Fax: -49-241-82455 Email: mbartneck@ukaachen.de

1. NANOMEDICINES AND THERANOSTICS

1.1. Putative Anti-cancer Nanomedicines and their Biodistribtion

Nanomedicines, nanotechnologically generated drugs, cover a broad range of sizes of a few up to several hundred nanometers [1]. Depending on the nature of the material, they can be classified into two major groups, organic or inorganic. In many cases, the organic particulates are clinically usable and the inorganic formulations are mostly used in research. Gold nanoparticles (AuNP) probably are the most intensively studied type of inorganic nanoparticle. AuNP can easily be altered in terms of size, shape, and functionalization such as nanorods [2], nanocages [3], or nanostars [4]. The metallic nature allows for optical and magnetic properties to be traced in whole body-based and cellular imaging [5, 6]. However, a drawback of inorganic nanoparticles is given by their temporal accumulation in the body, owed to their missing degradability. Earlier own studies have demonstrated that gold nanorods reside in the liver to a similar extent after seven days compared to the level after one day [5]. Importantly, not all organic nanoparticles, for instance fullerenes or carbon nanotubes [7], are biodegradable.

A huge number of organic nanoparticles have been generated. Importantly, liposomes and the particles based on polymers such as N-(2-Hydroxypropyl) methacrylamide (HPMA) belong to the most successful formulations [8]. Most organic nanoparticles exhibit the major advantage of being biodegradable by means of their composition. For instance, liposomes can be integrated into the cell membrane which also contain phospholipids or cholesterol [9]. Most nanoparticles, in particular AuNP [5], but also iron oxide-based formulations, are non-toxic at clinically usable concentrations [10]. Importantly, very small AuNP of size 1.4 nm are toxic to cells [11]. Nevertheless, the dose determines the toxicity and at high doses, many nanotherapeutics can be toxic as demonstrated for titanium dioxide nanoparticles [12]. Certain materials can be toxic, *i.e.* silica-based nanoparticles exhibit immunotoxicity by activating macrophages [13, 14]. To reduce the adherence of serum proteins to therapeutics, PEGylation, the decoration with a PEG layer, is carried out to reduce the unspecific internalization by phagocytes based on a neutral charge which repels many types of proteins [15]. Specific functionalizations, such as peptides [16], can affect an immune response, such as that of macrophages and dendritic cells [5, 16, 17].

Liposomal formulations are the most successful ones, based on their market size. Novel formulations continuously enter the market and recently, Vyxeos gained approval for the treatment of acute myeloid leukemia (AML) in August 2017. Vyxeos delivers both cytarabine and daunorubicin at a molar ratio of 5:1 [18]. Vyxeos showed an improvement in the efficacy in two phase 2 clinical trials, compared with a standard cytarabine and daunorubicin regimen [19, 20].

Promising novel clinical trials are those on drugs with a temperature-inducible drug release, specifically Thermodox (Celsion Corp.) [21]. This liposomal doxorubicin is prepared with thermally sensitive lipids that degrade on exposure to high heat and disrupt the lipid bilayer, evoking drug release [21, 22]. The combination of nanodrug with radiofrequency thermal ablation allows the drug to be released in a site-specific manner at the tumor [21, 22]. Many clinical trials in phase 3 on combined Thermodox and radiofrequency ablation technique have been completed or are still in progress [22].

Polymers can be natural, synthetic, or pseudosynthetic [23]. Polyethylene glycol (PEG) is the most frequently used polymer [21]. Polymeric nanomedicines form an important pillar in nanomedicine since many studies have reported their high efficacy, safety, and prolonged drug release [21, 24]. As a result, polymeric NPs seem to be promising nano-carriers for various medications [24]. Polymeric NPs can be formulated by adding agents to their surface that can be utilized in diagnostic imaging [24]. Biodegradable polymers have attracted the attention of many researchers in recent years since they can be completely metabolized and thus removed from the body [24]. PLGA (polylactic-glycolic acid) is an interesting biodegradable polymer based on its relative proportions of polylactic acid (PLA) and polyglycolic acid. The ratio between both constituents can be used to modulate the biodegradability behavior of PLGA [24].

Micelles are self-assembling polymeric NPs with a hydrophobic internal core used to encapsulate drugs that have a low degree of solubility in aqueous solution, while the external surface of a micelle has enough polarity to allow dissolution in aqueous media [21]. The drugs delivered by micelles include many hydrophobic drugs, including anti-cancer medicines [25 - 28]. Polymeric micelles can deliver their cargo using both passive and active targeting capabilities. Active targeting of specific receptors can enhance the selectivity of drug delivery and thus potentially decreases the side effects [29]. For tumor targeting, micellar NPs utilize the so-called enhanced permeability and retention (EPR) effect [30, 31] for passive accumulation, while they make use of certain ligands, such as antibodies or folic acid [32] for deliberate active targeting. Stealth micelles sizing 10–100 nm are large enough to avoid excretion through the kidneys, and at the same time they are sufficiently small to overcome filtration in the spleen. In sum, this leads to a prolonged circulation time of these particles [33]. Therefore, polymeric micelles enable a directed delivery of higher drug doses to target sites while reducing systemic toxicity [32].

Micelle-based Estrasorb is FDA approved for vasomotor-associated symptoms during with menopause [21]. The delivery of Estrasorb allows high concentrations of drug through the skin which in turn reduces contact with the gastrointestinal tract and also a reduced hepatic first-pass effect [34] thereby enabling stable serum levels for 8 to 14 days which is desired since this reduces repeated administration [21]. Nanoplatin, micellar cisplatin, is currently evaluated in phase 2 trials as single drug or in combination with other chemotherapeutics (for instance, gemcitabine). On the other hand, two phase 1 clinical trials of a micellar nano-form of SN-38, an active metabolite of the topo-isomerase inhibitor irinotecan, have been completed. Further, phase 2 trials on solid tumors, NSCLC, and triple-negative breast cancer have also been carried out. In addition, Genexol-PM (mPEG-block-D, L-PLA micellar paclitaxel), is being developed as a substitute for Kolliphor-based paclitaxel [22]. Several phase 1–2 trials were completed in metastatic breast cancer or NSCLC patients [35 - 37].

Dendrimers are polymeric macromolecules designed in a branched manner with a surface susceptible to be modified with desired functional groups. This unique configuration attracts researchers to use them as drug [38, 39] and gene [40 - 42] delivery systems. In addition, the dendrimers' architecture allows the active pharmacological materials to be encapsulated in the central core or bound to the surface by electrostatic or hydrophobic interactions [43]. A variety of dendrimers were generated. Polyamidoamine (PAMAM)-derived dendrimers are the most successful and applicable ones and are favorable for drug delivery owed to their hydrophilicity, biocompatibility, and non-immunogenicity [44 - 48]. Also, Poly-L-lysine (PLL) dendrimers [49 - 51] are characterized by high biocompatibility and biodegradability. Drugs can be encapsulated within the dendrimer NPs based on chemical and physical interactions [52]. Physical interactions control the entrapment of the drug within the interior cavity of the particle by certain types of noncovalent binding, such as hydrogen bonds, electrostatic interactions, or hydrophobic forces. The central core of dendrimer NPs is mostly hydrophobic; thus, it encapsulates the hydrophobic drugs. Concerning the chemical interactions, they include covalent binding of the drugs with functional desired moieties of the dendrimer NPs and they exhibit a high stability [53, 54].

The surface of PAMAM dendrimer NPs has high susceptibility for several modifications to achieve an improved type of cancer therapy. Active targeting is one of approaches used to deliver the cargo to the targeted site to increase the tumor specificity and decrease systemic toxicity [55]. In such approach, antibodies can be used to specify the targeted tumor and release the cargo to the correct area. Based on the active targeting strategy, Kulhari *et al.* [56] established a G4 dendrimer NPs encapsulating docetaxel (DTX). The particles were further surface modified with trastuzumab (TZ) and PEG was used as a linker. TZ is applicable for immunotherapy of those types of cancer that express elevated levels of the human epidermal growth factor receptor type 2 (HER2) [57]. Kulharis' research team investigated the *in vitro* efficacy of the TZ-DTX-dendrimers as compared to DTX-dendrimers and frees DTX by cultivation with HER2-positive and HER2-negative cells. The TZ-DTX-dendrimer was taken up to a significantly larger extent than the DTX-dendrimer, whereas no difference was observed in HER-negative cells. The cytotoxicity of the modified dendrimer accordingly also was higher in HER-positive cells. The IC_{50} concentration of the TZ-DTX-dendrimer was 3.6-times higher than that of the DTX-dendrimer, and no difference noted between each of them or the free drug in HER-negative cells [56].

Regardless of the approval of the rising number of nanoparticle-based formulations approved for cancer treatment, dendrimers did not undergo FDA approval yet.

Iron oxide NPs have been studied in various clinical trials investigating their use as contrast reagent for magnetic resonance imaging (MRI) [22]. However, the majority of FDA-approved iron oxide nanodrugs are indicated as iron-replacement therapies [58 - 60]. Utilizing iron oxide NPs aims to increase the concentration of iron in the body [61]. Such approaches have to be intensively investigated to estimate the toxicity levels associated with the injection of free iron [59, 60], taking into consideration the harmful effects of *in vitro* and *in vivo* due to the generation of reactive oxygen species [62]. Macdougall and Danielson have reported that using sugars to coat colloidal iron might help to get rid of these toxicity issues [59, 60].

The unique features of gold NPs allow them to be used as a promising tool not only for cancer diagnosis but also for drug delivery applications. Moreover, gold nanoparticles exhibit a non-toxic and non-immunogenic nature. Gold NPs have demonstrated promising results as antineoplastic agents when used either individually or as a drug delivery vector [22]. Preclinical studies using gold NPs as a drug delivery vector to deliver tumor necrosis factor alpha (TNFα) have shown a reduction in the toxicity rates; however, they indicated with low clinical value because of their rapid clearance by the reticuloendothelial system. To tackle this challenge, gold NPs were conjugated with PEG moiety which significantly prolonged their half-life time in the blood [22]. Aurimune (CYT-6091), a PEG-gold N, has been used as a vector to transmit recombinant tumor necrosis factor alpha into tumors. It was reported that Aurimune was tolerated well by patients with advanced cancer [63]. Moreover, the PEG layer reduces the uptake by the mononuclear phagocyte system (MPS) which in turn enhances the drug accumulation within the tumor *via* the EPR effect [63]. This first phase trial was successfully completed reporting a safe delivery of TNF which is intended to effectively kill cancer cells [63].

Currently, researchers are focusing on both, *in vivo* bio-distribution, and photothermal applications of gold NP which are related to their unique ability to absorb near infrared (NIR)-light [64]. Aurolase®, PEG-silica-gold nanoshells, were developed for thermal ablation of solid tumors following NIR light induction leading to thermal tumor melting [65]. However, clinical trials with Aurolase were not completed (trials NCT01679470), and side effects were noted (trial NCT00848042) in patients with recurrent and/or refractory head and neck cancer.

A few AuNP-based theranostics have progressed into clinical trials. For instance, a current clinical study to investigate the safety issues of NU-0129, a gold-NP encapsulated small interfering RNA (siRNAs) against Bcl-2-like protein 12 (BCL2L12), has shown its antineoplastic activity in a phase I study (NCT03020017). Another study has been implemented clinically by Kharlamov and colleagues to determine the safety and efficacy of two different delivery methods for gold NPs for atherosclerosis therapy. The first is a photothermal therapy (PTT)-based approach that makes use of silica-gold hybrid NP. The second one is a magnetic-assisted navigation strategy facilitating silica-gold iron bearing NPs (NCT01270139) [66]. This trial reported that the PTT approach utilizing gold-silica NPs declined the coronary atherosclerosis significantly with more tolerability and safety for the clinical use. Also, an ongoing clinical study to include breath analysis using a nano-sensor array to recognize gastric diseases is ongoing (NCT01420588). Researchers speculate that the nano-sensor array may represent an urgently needed non-invasive screening method to distinguish gastric cancer from other related precancerous lesions [67].

Many different parameters such as material type, size range, and functionalization affect the distribution in different cells and organs. It is assumed that the size is the most important parameter of nanoparticles for their interaction with cells and tissues. A study has demonstrated that of AuNP which sizing either 10, 50, 100, or 250 nm, most gold was found in liver and spleen for particles above 50 nm. The nanoparticles that were smaller than 10 nm were found to be distributed widespread to many other organs such as kidney, testis, and brain [68]. We have observed before that accumulation in liver and spleen also is apparent for gold nanorods sizing 50x15 nm [5]. The liver has an exceptional capacity for nanoparticle clearance which can be explained by its huge size (the largest internal organ of the body) compared to the spleen. In fact, the dry weight of the liver is approximately 50-fold higher than that of the spleen [5].

The organ distribution of magnetic iron oxide-based nanoparticles is similar to that of AuNP. For instance, it was observed that iron oxide-based NP with a core size of 11 nm distribute at similar amounts in different organs in the body [10]. However, also chemicals such as the polymer polyethylene glycol (PEG) which stabilizes NP can accumulate in the liver after particle destabilization. The strong accumulation of nanoparticles larger than 50 nm in the liver renders them ideal candidates for targeting liver diseases when used for drug delivery. However, this also puts them into the focus of many other types of therapies in which liver accumulation actually is not wanted [69].

1.2. Theranostic Medicines

Theranostics comprise in many cases medical applications that are imaging-guided so that the drug or the carrier can be traced in diagnostics [70]. The tracing strategies in theranostics depend on the possibilities for detecting particles in cells and on the whole organism level. Non-fluorescent components such as lipid or polymeric shells can get detectable *in vivo* by using integratable fluorescent tags, *i.e.* 1,2-dioleoyl-sn-glycero-3-phosphoethanolamine-N-(7-nitro-2-1,3-benzoxadi-azol-4-yl) (NBD-PE) [9]. Of the inorganic nanoparticles, particularly the metal-based ones such as gold nanoparticles, can be detected in computerized tomography owed to their electron density nanomedicines further enable regional and controlled delivery of the encapsulated drug. The immune system represents an important interactor for nanotheranostics, with both cells and the factors in body fluids. Particularly, the process of immune-related molecules binding to foreign material that is called opsonization also critically accounts for nanomaterials. Importantly, serum proteins bind to particulate or implant materials and act as important opsonins. The first and most successful theranostic drug is available for treatment of pancreatic and gastrointestinal neuroendocrine tumors (carcinoids). In general, these tumors grow slowly and are metastatic at the time of diagnosis. The tumors can treated with somatostatin analogs, such as octreotide and lanreotide, what leads to a reduction in the hormonal overproduction of the tumors [71].

In the 1990s, the so-called peptide-receptor radionuclide therapy (PRRT) that makes use of radiolabeled somatostatin analogs was introduced as an innovative treatment option for patients with inoperable gastroenteropancreatic neuroendocrine tumors. The treatment is based on the fact that the majority of these tumors express elevated levels of the somatostatin receptor. This increased expression can be studied in whole body imaging by using somatostatin analogues such as radiolabeled somatostatin analog, ^{111}In-diethylenetriamine pentaacetic acid (DTPA)-octreotide. Based on the identification of these tumors by the octreotide, a strategy for active targeting was developed [71]. With molecular weights of 1019 Da for octreotide and 1096 Da for lanreotide, these analogues are almost in the size range of small molecules which usually range until 800 Da.

Radiolabeled analogs of somatostatin are represented by three main constituents: a cyclic octapeptide (*i.e.* Tyr3-octreotide/Tyr3-octreotate), a chelating agent (for instance, DTPA or tetraazacyclododecane tetraacetic acid, DOTA), and a radioactive tracer. Radioisotopes that are commonly used in PRRT are 111In, ^{90}Y, and ^{177}Lu. A recent review outlined that ^{177}Lu-octreotate, which belongs to the third generation of somatostatin-receptor-directed radionuclids, results in stable disease in 35% of patients and in tumor remission for 46% of patients. Further, a survival benefit of several years was identified [71].

1.3. Nanomedicines for Passive and Active Targeting

Nanomedicines have significantly advanced the field of drug delivery [22]. Some key novelties of nanomedicines are active and passive targeting, as well as "smart" behavior. While passive targeting represents the way of action of the currently approved nanomedicines such as Doxil, the concept of nanoparticle-facilitated cell targeting continuously raises the interest of scientists. One example for the over-appreciation of active targeting is the prostate-specific membrane antigen targeted nanocarrier for docetaxel, BIND-014. It did not achieve the anticipated success since it was not superior over non-targeted liposomal formulations [27]. The option to combine different drugs represents another great promise of nanomedicine: for instance, the liposomal drug CPX-351 includes two different chemotherapeutics and has entered phase III trials with excellent response rates in patients with acute myeloid lymphoma, based on using synergistic effects of different components [28]. This suggests that combinatory nanomedicines based on liposomal formulations are rather suitable to advance therapeutics than ligands for cell type-specific targeting [29].

The nanotechnological tools allow for a huge variety of concepts and can be composed of diverse biological units: *i.e.*carbohydrates, proteins, lipids, and nucleic acids. Carbohydrates are vital to energy saving and also are parts of glycoproteins. NM can and have adopted several miniaturizations from larger macromolecules. For instance, functional sugar carbohydrate groups of larger glycoproteins can be used separately from their protein part. We have demonstrated before that selectins (glycoproteins), can be reduced to their carbohydrate part and their biological functionality still remains functional [72]. We have recently analyzed the efficiency of selectin-binding glycoproteins. We found that a certain construct was able to inhibit the migration of human primary MΦ based on the carbohydrate part only [72]. Furthermore, it exhibited therapeutic effects for inflammatory liver disease by acting on macrophages in the liver (Kupffer cells) [73].

Lipid-based drugs are an important transport vehicle, and have demonstrated long-term success for instance in chemotherapeutics. Lipids and particularly phospholipids are useful to design fully biocompatible drug delivery systems [9, 74], or parts of the membranes of artificial cells. Using lipids for drug encapsulation dramatically changes the pharmacokinetics of drugs such as the significantly increased circulation of doxorubicin, pioneered by Gabizon and colleagues in the 1990s [75], a method allowing for the enhanced permeability and retention (EPR) effect of NM [76].

Miniaturization of protein domains or other motifs is a common strategy in nanomedicines design. The tripeptide arginine-glycine-asparagine (RGD) probably is the most frequently used and most intensively studied bioactive peptide. It is derived from the protein Fibronectin and other proteins of the extracellular matrix and sizes 350 Da only Similar to the Fibronectin, RGD binds to integrin motifs at the cell surface and thereby mediates attachment of many cell types. Thereby, it enables attachment of cells to PEG which otherwise cannot attach to them. *I.e.* cell-repellant materials such as PEGylated, poly acrylic acid (PAA)-coated, or fluorinated and hydrophobic substrates can thus be decorated with RGD and thereby mediate cellular attachment.

Ligands that are miniaturized motifs are interesting for equipping NM to evoke targeting specificity. In this regard, nanobodies and aptamers may enrich diverse microscopical and imaging methods, *i.e.* by enhanced resolution [77]. Nanobodies size 2 to 4 nm and exhibit a molecular weight of about 12-15 kDa and are made of 100-120 amino acids [77]. They contain the part of antibodies which binds selectively. Aptamers exhibit the advantage compared to conventional proteins and antibody-based targeting by being less instable and more sensitive than proteins. They are chemically produced based on self-folding oligonucleotides with 15–100 nucleotides [78] sizing 2-3 nm and weighing 10 to 15 kDa. Size reductions represent a great advantage in microscopical and imaging methods, since some small antigens offer as few as ten binding sites [77]. In contrast to their minimized versions, many natural antibodies have a molecular weight of 50-200 kDa and a size of approximately 10 nm [79].

Nanomedicines can adapt smart features by specific modifications. The first approved NM was liposomal doxorubicine (Doxil®) which received FDA approval in 1995. Doxil targeted passively to tumors and makes use of the EPR effect. Yet, the release of its cargo is based on a yet unknown mechanism [80]. Increasing drug release is a key strategy for enhancing its performance and the specific conditions of diseased sites which affect temperature and pH can be used for NM drug design. Notably, the temperature increased in inflammation, particularly during fever [81]. In wounds [82], and in the skin [82], the pH is below seven which is considered as acidic pH. Consequential, NM should be generated in a way that they allow for controlled release at the desired region (organ or tissue) facilitated, for example through temperature and pH-induced physiological settings.

The observation of disease specific settings can virtually be extended much further. For instance, responsiveness can be achieved towards redox potential, as well [83], or towards enzymes which catalyze a specific reaction near the pathogenic lesion [84]. Furthermore, smart features can be electric pulse-sensitive, photosensitive, or magnetic field-sensitive [85]. Gel-based systems may further amplify the options of materials, *i.e.* mediated by swelling behavior and a potential interactive drug release [86]. Many NM-based drugs act intracellulary and thus have to be delivered into the cytoplasm. In the ideal case, a smart material feature can make use of a certain mechanism to assure endosomal escape [87]. The cargo, *i.e.* a nucleic acid, has to get out of the carrier before it is degraded by enzymes of the lysosome which form in late endosomes. Endosomal escape can for instance be realized *via* incorporation of pH-sensitive lipids, leading to enhanced release of nucleic acids in lysosomal regions where the pH is low [88].

In summary, the exploitation of smart features represents a key step in overcoming biological carriers and to enable controlled drug release, particularly of nucleic acid-based drugs.

1.4. How Omics Data can be Used to Develop Improved (nano-) Drugs

The sequencing of the human genome in 2000 has led to tremendous efforts to further understand the dynamics of DNA in genomics and of RNA in transcriptomics. Nucleic acids keep and transmit the genetic information. In the 1950s, DNA was identified as the keeper of genetic information and the classical dogma of molecular biology ever since was that this DNA can be transcribed into mRNA which can be translated into a functional protein. Omics are the collection of techniques used to characterize and quantify pools of biological molecules and to explore their roles, relationships and actions within an organism. The Omics technologies utilize high-throughput (HT) methods to generate what is today referred to as big data. Computer-aided data mining is required to enable improved understanding of correlations and dependencies in disease. The age of systems medicine has led to the identification of pathological networks, consequences of mutations in the genetic code, and connected signaling pathways from different sections of human biology. Therefore, linked analysis of data obtained from genomics, transcriptomics, metabolomics, and proteomics are functionally linked, and deciphering these links represents a key issue of systems medicine.

In case of diseases that are attributable to a genetic mutation, the mutated alleles represent potential biomarker that might aid in the identification of an appropriate patient population. Precision medicine at the bedside may employ proteins causative for the inherited disease. The Omics-based technologies are integer parts during all all phases of pharmaceutical drug development. The integration of genetic and protein-associated data enables to identify correlations between gene loci and protein dysfunction [89], thereby enabling to identify novel attempts for treatment.

Omics strongly helped oncology to transform from targeting aberrant pathways associated with mutated genes to gene therapy. The FDA has stated that in sum 18 small molecular drugs and biological-based drugs were approved for treating different types of cancer along with corresponding companion diagnostics. The small molecule-based tyrosine kinase inhibitor (TKI) imatinib was the first drug of these which was approved for chronic myeloid leukemia (CML). The approval of imatinib initiated a new chapter in targeted therapy.

The capabilities for curing cancer have recently been extended by gene therapy (CAR-T cell therapy). The current CAR-T cell therapies treat B-cell induced lymphoblastic leukemia: the autologous T cells of the patient are genetically modified to express chimeric antigen receptors that enable to specifically kill cancer cells.

The omics technologies provide a strong data background for improved precision nanomedicines. Owed to the fact that late stage drug development represents the most costly part of the process, the appropriate drug should be generated for the appropriate patient with the appropriate disease [90]. Omics technologies are an integral part of informed pharmaceutical R&D and their role in R&D will very likely expand further [90]. One major issue in integrating Omics data will be the establishment of omics data generation standards, aiming to reduce inter laboratory variability and to increase confidence in distinctly classifying disease subtypes to assist in the design of clinical trials.

We anticipate that the advances in omics will be a key issue for the upcoming collections of precision medicine. Tens of thousands of biomarkers (genomes, proteomes, transcriptomics, interactomes, microRNAomes, *etc.*) deliver information for keys periods of different types of diseases. In summary, application of omics technologies to ever-evolving biomedical innovations, such as disease-on-chip technologies, is the path towards personalized medicines. The generation of the respective big data sets and its efficient analysis, *i.e.* based on computer algorithms represents the key path to novel avenues in medicine.

1.5. Strategies to Localize Drug Delivery

The current practice in cancer treatment is still based on surgery, chemotherapy, and radiotherapy. However, these techniques exhibit only a moderate level of specificity since the cells of solid tumors may remain in the body. Thus, improved strategies very likely need to have high specificity, high efficacy, and low adverse effects. A local drug delivery thus remains an attractive perspective for cancer treatment. However, as a drawback, many nanomedicines frequently require repeated injections. Thus, there is a high need to develop drug delivery systems which release the drug at the target site. Controlled drug release of from nanomaterials thus is a hot topic in cancer therapy. Methods for preparation of NPs are most frequently given by so-called 'bottom-up' methods in which nanomaterials are generated from atoms or molecules in a thermodynamically controlled system organized by means such as self-assembly [91]. The NPs require specific properties which should work in a harmonic fashion to qualify them to reach and in the best case, even to remain in the targeted area. Those characters are combinations of material size, nature, and modifications. This further result in features such as surface chemistry, hydrophilicity/hydrophobicity, biodegradability, surface functionalization, and physical response properties (temperature, pH, electric charge, light, sound, magnetism). The corresponding drug delivery systems exhibit advantages from (i) the ability to target a specific region of space in the body; (ii) the reduced amount of drug quantity required to maintain a particular concentration at the target site; and (iii) reduced drug concentration at non-target sites [92] which minimizes side effects.

Magnetic drug delivery systems are a prominent approach for the delivery of various pharmacological agents to target specific area using engineered smart carriers. With the support of a magnetic field, the drug is precisely targeted towards the diseased area. The core-shell magnetic NPs which are frequently used for this purpose consist of metals or metal oxides cores encapsulated by a certain coating. The magnetic specifications of such particles enable their integration into different applications such as (i) magnetic contrast compounds which can be used *i.e.* for magnetic resonance imaging (MRI) [93]; (ii) hyperthermia enabling agents, which are heated by a high frequency magnetic field. (*e.g.* thermal ablation/tumor hyperthermia) [94]; and (iii) magnetic vectors which can be guided by means of a magnetic field gradient, thereby for instance enabling drug delivery [95].

Targeting of tumors hence can be done utilizing magnetic nanocarriers by passive strategies, or by active mechanisms. Passive targeting is among others based on the extravasation of the NPs in the tumor area where the microvasculature is hyperpermeable and leaky. Consequential NP accumulate at these regions that are located in tumor tissue, a phenomenon known as enhanced permeation and retention (EPR) effect [96]. Alternatively, targeting of tumors can be based on the active strategy, *i.e.* based on tumor-specific ligands. Yet, active targeting of tumors appears inapplicable because of the short residence time in the circulation in addition to the lower concentration of NP in the region where the tumor is located (despite the EPR effect) what frequently leads to drug concentrations below the therapeutic level and to off-target accumulation is frequently observed in active targeting approaches [30].

Magnetic liposomes (magnetosomes) can be prepared by (a) incorporation of magnetic particles in the phospholipid linkage which acts as nanoreactor while in second method (b) phosphatidylcholine/phosphatidylethanolamine are used in the 2:1 ratio covering the magnetic particles, which produces agglomerates of the magnetic particles. Magnetosomes are advantageous because of their ability to easily escape from the reticuloendothelial system, *i.e.* based on the PEGylation of liposomes, thus enabling exploitation of their sensitivity towards the magnetic field [97].

Unfortunately, there are many factors which remain barriers for the clinical use of magnetic drug delivery. The main factor which limits the use of magnetic NPs in drug delivery is the required high strength of a magnetic field that is needed to direct the NPs in the blood stream to accumulate at targeted area or to trigger the drug release. To avoid these issues, internal magnets can be implanted in the area nearby the target site using a precise small surgery. Many studies have identified a reasonable targeted drug delivery using magnetic implants [98, 99].

Drug delivery systems can be responsive towards various different stimuli, such as pH [100, 101], temperature [102, 103], and enzymes [104 - 107]. Yet, this triggered drug release relies on the specific properties of the *in vivo* environments. Particularly light responsive systems have received great attention related to the opportunity for spatial (and temporal) resolution [108 - 112]. The key mechanism in photo-controlled drug delivery systems is the light-induced transformation of the respective light responsive molecules that in turn undergo conformational changes, *i.e.* degradation, phase change, and more, what consequentially triggers drug release. In general, ultraviolet (UV) and visible (vis) light can be used in this regard to trigger the response of the material based on the energy transition of photons [113 - 117]. However, key limitations of light-induced systems are low tissue penetration and putative tissue damage, frequently causing difficulties *in vivo* [113]. One option to solve these issues is to shift the "biological transparency window" towards the near-infrared (NIR) region between 650 to 900 nm of wavelength. Light scattering and absorption are minimized at this region, thereby enabling greater tissue penetration depth than UV and vis lights [115, 118 - 121].

However, also NIR light is limited to about 10 mm penetration depth into tissue.

During the past decades, numerous nanocarriers, including liposomes [122, 123], polymers [124 - 127], and dendrimers [128 - 130] have been used to deliver drugs to tumors in the course of chemotherapy. Further, mesoporous silica nanoparticles (MSNs) have been explored that exhibit a large surface area and a large pore volume for loading with drugs, as well as the option to be functionalized [129, 131 - 137]. Particularly the pores offer the possibility to be functionalized with light responsive chemicals and organic switch molecules that render the MSNs into light responsive drug delivery systems.

NIR-triggered drug delivery of MSN has in the past been achieved by two main principles: lanthanide doped up-conversion particles (UCNPs), that enable a transfer of NIR light into UV/vis radiation [138 - 140], and particles that convert NIR light into thermal signals. Several different particles exhibit this opportunity, for instance, precious metal based particles with NIR plasma resonance, carbon based materials, semiconductor nanocrystals with NIR absorption, and many others [141 - 146]. Solely inorganic nanoparticles mentioned above generally exhibit the drawbacks of low biocompatibility and low drug loading capacity. These limitations apparently suit well to the advantages of MSNs. Due to limitations in the efficiency of NIR-responsive nanomaterials, the functional polymers are needed to be very sensitive to stimuli and thus these toggles must be carefully selected. The combination of these different materials for NIR-triggered drug delivery systems is a simple type of designing and fabricating smart-functioning nano-bots [147 - 151].

In NIR light-triggered uncaging of active substances from the mesopores of the UCNP-mSiO$_2$ hybrid nanoparticles, drug release is inhibited by crosslinked photosensitive molecules that shield the mesopores. Following irradiation with NIR light, doped UCNPs transform NIR photons into photon of the UV/vis spectrum. The process is followed by the dissociation of the light responsive molecular porters, thereby, "opening" the mesopore "gates", thereby enabling drug release. Multiple different photo-responsive (labile) molecules were developed for this process [152, 153]. Particularly nitrobenzyl (NB) and some derivatives have been used extensively as photo-labile groups that function as "caging" molecules [154]. Yang and colleagues conjugated NB with long-chain oligo(ethylene) glycol in order to function as cage linkers. They demonstrated NIR light-triggered liberation of doxorubicin (DOX) from UCNP@mSiO$_2$ hybrid nanoparticles. Furthermore, they linked amino-functionalized cationic NB siRNA which is anionic, and attached the construct onto the surface of the UCNP@SiO$_2$ particles. This design enabled a controlled cleavage and release of the siRNA from the particles as induced by radiation with 980 nm NIR [155]. Jayakumar and coworkers have also developed a system for controlled release of siRNAs and plasmid DNA from UCNP@mSiO$_2$ NP. In their study, caging was achieved with 4,5-dimethoxy-2-nitroacetophenone (DMNPE). The exposure of NIR light triggered gene expression in their study [156]. The above mentioned NIR responsive nucleic acid delivery systems have demonstrated that controllable NIR-induced drug release is feasible and they further reduced the side effects of the system, particularly photo-damage.

1.6. Therapeutic Options of Small Non-coding RNA

During the beginning of this century, small non-coding RNA (sncRNA) was discovered. SncRNA includes *i.e.* small interfering RNA (siRNA) and micro-RNAs (miR) exhibit enzymatic functions that enable the modulation of gene activity. The widely used siRNA is specific for inhibiting one specific target mRNA which is normally translated into a protein. On the contrary, miR can up and down-regulate multiple different targets in transcription and translation [157].

Bioinformatics science has demonstrated that about 60% of protein coding genes are regulated by miR [158]. The mechanism of action of miR is facilitated through binding to the 3' untranslated region of one or several target mRNA(s). The generally low specificity of miR is a consequence of the fact that it just binds partially to mRNA. Consequential, few miR can bind to only one target, while it is more common that they bind to multiple different targets [159]. MiR is critically involved into the regulation of inflammatory liver disease, as outlined by Roy and colleagues [160]. Therefore, a modulation of miR activity represents an efficient means to overcome disease processes in inflammatory diseases and cancer.

One of the great pioneers in developing nanomedicines for nucleic acid development is Pieter Cullis (University of British Columbia in Vancouver, Canada). He stated that a third generation of nanomedicines is on the run: those that shuttle molecules such as RNA which are much more difficult to deliver than small molecules [161]. Further exploiting the potential of miR exhibits a huge and unique therapeutic potential. Intracellular processing of miR starts in the nucleus from where primary miR (pri-miR) is transferred to the cytoplasm. The precursor miR (pre-miR) is further processed into a guide and a passenger strand by the enzyme DICER. Synthetic miR modulators such as pro-miR (to induce) or anti-miR (to inhibit) are capable of regulating endogenous mature (guide strand) miR (Fig. **1**).

Notably, the toxicity, immunogenicity, and instability of sncRNA in circulation require strategies to facilitate efficient delivery to target sites, [162] and the poor delivery remains the limiting factor for clinical translation [159]. Generally, there are viral and non-viral delivery systems for snc RNA. The viral vectors have the drawbacks of immunogenicity, mutagenesis, and high costs. Consequently, non-viral delivery systems employing mainly lipids or polymers are most popular [159, 162]. The most widely used vector for sncRNA delivery is lipoplexes which consist of randomly formed complexes of cationic lipids and the negatively charged sncRNA. However, lipoplexes exhibit toxic effects due to their strong positive charge [163], which omits their use in the clinics. Lipid-based drug with neutral surface charge are ideal vectors for sncRNA because the most successful nanomedicines such as Doxil™/Caelyx™ are PEGylated liposomal formulations. In line with the historical developments, most of the novel miR therapeutics which are at clinical trials target cancer.

Very recently, the first drug based on a siRNA has been approved: ONPATTRO™ (patisiran), which was developed by Alnylam Pharmaceuticals. It is tailored to treat the polyneuropathy that is a consequence of hereditary Transthyretin-mediated amyloidosis. ONPATTRO™ is composed of a double-stranded siRNA that is encapsulated in a lipid capsule. The lipid formulation evokes delivery to hepatocytes which then do no longer produce the pathogenic protein. Patisiran has recently also been approved for the treatment of the polyneuropathy induced by hereditary TTR-mediated amyloidosis (hATTR) in adults in the USA and subsequently and it was also approved by the EMA for the treatment of hATTR in adults for stage 1 or 2 of the polyneuropathy [164].

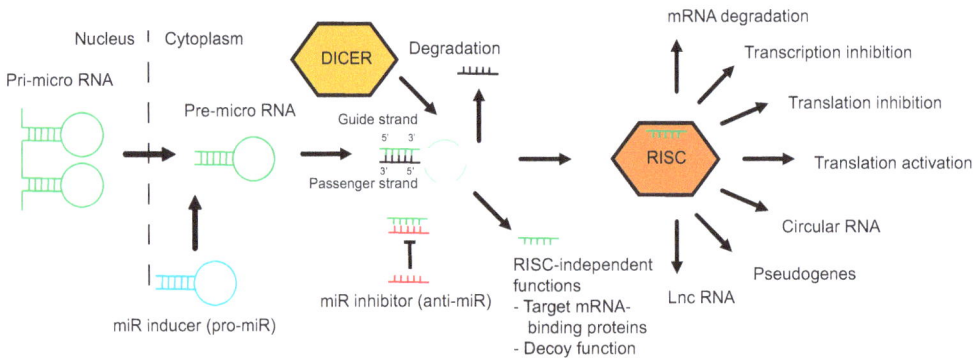

Fig. (1). Intracellular micro-RNA processing and targets of the RISC. There are two basic ways of modulating miR by miR modulators. Pre/pro-miR can induce the expression of a certain endogenous miR and thereby switch on certain proteins. The DICER enzyme plays an important role in processing the miR, while the combination of RISC and guide strand miR perform the corresponding enzymatic activities based on partial base pairing.

2. IMMUNE CELL-DIRECTED THERAPIES

2.1. Lymphoid Cells are in the Focus of Cancer Therapy

Leukocytes exhibit a unique level of mobility and are able to reach nearly any part of the human body. While every organ contains specific specialized cell types such as the hepatocytes or the liver, leukocytes of different organs share several similarities [5]. Basically, one can differentiate lymphoid *versus* myeloid immune cells. Further decipheration of three main types of lymphocytes can be done: natural killer (NK) cells, B lymphocytes, and T lymphocytes. The innate NK cells perform important functions in killing abnormal or cancer cells that lack MHC I markers on their surface and that are therefore considered as abnormal. T and B lymphocytes are specific towards a single antigen only and can be activated by antigen-presenting cells such as macrophages. Targeting of the lymphoid cells can be done using monoclonal antibodies against surface markers that are specific for a certain cell population. The monoclonal antibody rituximab which depletes $CD20^+$ cells (B cells) was FDA-approved in 1998 for B cell lymphoma and was the first antibody approved for cancer therapy. Monoclonal (monospecific) antibodies such as rituximab act by setting a label to a designated cell type which can then readily be eliminated by by other immune cells which recognize the Fc-part of the antibody. During the last decade, bispecific antibodies have been employed to further enhance the therapeutic capabilities of therapeutic antibodies by binding and thereby functionally connecting two different binding sites.

Improving the efficiency of monoclonal antibodies can be achieved by bispecific antibodies, conjugated antibodies that have two parts for specific binding and which can bind to two different targets on a single cell. Bispecific antibodies with affinity to both CD20 and FAS were developed. The surface marker CD20 is intended to target malignant B cells whereas FAS (CD95) is known to trigger apoptosis by binding to the FAS ligand. Interestingly, the sole binding of FAS only is not efficient to induce apoptosis [165]. Thus, CD20×CD95 antibodies and similar conjugated might open new avenues for treating B-cell-mediated autoimmune disease and lymphoma [166].

The cytotoxic T cells have the capability to selectively eliminate cancer cells that express a specific surface antigen in the setting of anti-PD1 cancer immunotherapy. Through using an antibody against PD1, PDL1, or CTLA-4, the capability of CD8 cells to kill cancer cells is greatly enhanced [167]. However, during autoimmune disease, they are over reactive and can destroy the cells of the own body. Consequentially, it is a therapeutic strategy to deplete CD8 cells in autoimmune disease [168]. The CAR T cell therapy similarly exploits the specificity of CD8+ T cells. The first CAR T cell therapy has been approved in

2017 by the FDA and it targets children and young adults with refractory or relapsed acute B-cell lymphoblastic leukemia [169]. CAR T cells are generated based on extracting and genetically engineering patient's immune cells *ex vivo*. The cells are later re-injected into the same patient where they eliminate cancer cells that express a specific antigen [170].

The regulatory T cells (T_{reg}) exhibit the capability to suppress several other immune cells, particularly by their secretion of interleukin 10 (IL10). Thus, also T_{regs} have become one focus of immunotherapies. In inflammatory disease of the ear, the inflammatory reaction is prolonged when T_{reg} are eliminated by a CD25 depleting antibody [171]. These data underline their importance in suppressing immunity, which is a key aim in treating inflammatory diseases.

Unfortunately, there were tragic episodes in earlier attempts to engage T cells. One example is given by the drug JCAR015 developed by Juno Therapeutics. It failed in treating acute B cell lymphoblastic leukemia because it led to excess fluids in the brains of patients. It has then been suspended in 2015 (trial NCT02535364). Similarly, in 2006, a superagonist of CD28 was used (TGN1412), which caused serious sickness within minutes of six people. Nevertheless, therapies engaging CD28 have been successful in arthritis therapy [172]. In summary, it is therefore important to remember for future developments that immunotherapies bear risks, and specifically that hyperactivation of T cells can lead to fatal consequences.

2.2. Evolving Therapies Targeting Macrophages and Other Myeloid Cells

One key factor for the strong translocation of nanoparticles into the liver can be led back to the strong presence of macrophages, approximately accounting for 80-90% of all macrophages of the body [173]. However, also neutrophils are of importance for liver diseases progression, based on their huge numbers, and by their production of reactive oxygen species and extracellular traps. In addition to their sizes, nanoparticle charge represents a key factor for their interactions with immune cells. We have demonstrated before that positive charges increase uptake by immune cells and endothelial cells [16]. The extracellular interactions of nanoparticles with immune cell secreted extracellular traps are similarly affected by the charge of the particles [174]. We have recently summarized some novel therapeutic concepts and targets for neutrophils in inflammatory disease, where we also highlight the interactions between neutrophils and macrophages [175].

In contrast to B and T lymphocytes, which actively manipulate their own DNA and proliferate based on clonal expansion; myeloid cells such as MΦ exhibit a high level of plasticity strongly reflected by changes in their mRNA expression profiles [176]. Macrophages can be polarized by diverse stimuli into many different specialized subpopulations. In contract to lymphocytes and in contrast to murine ones, human MΦ does not proliferate. Despite this fact, many studies that are based on mouse experiments only lead to the notion that also human macrophages are proliferative [177]. These "big eaters" are heavily impacted by their microenvironment that predestines different subpopulations based on gene expression, cell surface markers, and a certain secretion of cytokines [178]. The most important classification in MΦ dichotomy is the decipheration into inflammatory macrophages (M1-MΦ) or anti-inflammatory M2-MΦ, referring to their expression of various mediators and surface markers [15]. The is a natural balance and coexistence of macrophage subtypes. Outbalances between M1 and M2 can lead to diseases: M1-MΦ can be drivers of inflammatory diseases and were also reported to exhibit anti-tumoral activity, while M2-MΦ support tumor growth, yet also down-regulate inflammation and further support wound healing.

There is evidence that cancerogenesis is influenced by different MΦ subsets, but the role of the subsets not fully understood. Several reports demonstrated that M2-polarized MΦ is present in large numbers in cancer [179]. These can be designated as type 2 tumor-associated macrophages (TAM2). The TAM2 and other immune cells share immunosuppressive functions. For instance, also myeloid-derived suppressor cells, T helper 2 (Th2) cells, and T_{reg} secrete immunosuppressive cytokines such as IL10 and thereby allow for immune evasion of tumors [179, 180]. Depending on the detailed mode of activation, M2-MΦ produces other cytokines with anti-inflammatory effects. For instance, the CC chemokine ligand 18 (CCL18), transforming growth factor β (TGF-β), or interleukin 1 receptor antagonist (IL1RA) fall into this category [181]. Our recently published research on experimental liver cancer demonstrated that, in addition to the TAM2, there are also inflammatory TAM, which one might term as TAM1, which are highly distinctive from the TAM2 and from MDSC in mRNA profiles [179]. Moreover, the production of proangiogenic factors, particularly of the vascular endothelial growth factor (Vegf) suggests an important role of monocytes in angiogenesis. We have demonstrated that the inflammatory monocytes which infiltrate the liver upon injury express Vegfa which induces the formation of novel blood vessels [182]. It is obvious that the scheme shown in Fig. (**2**) is just an excerpt of few aspects of the roles of macrophages cancer. There are indeed several exceptions and additional specifications from the simplified scheme, for instance leukemia is mainly driven by the proliferation of a certain immune cell (Fig. **2**).

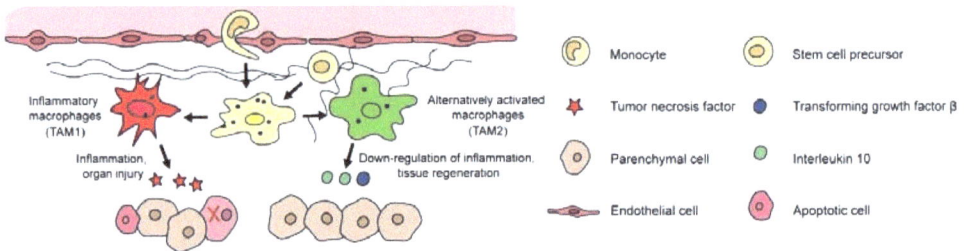

Fig. (2). Role of macrophage subpopulations in inflammatory disease and cancer. MΦ originate from bone marrow-derived circulating monocytes which migrate into injured organs *via* the bloodstream, and from local stem cells of the organ they reside. MΦ exhibit a unique level of plasticity, and the microenvironment can polarize them towards a plethora of subtypes including inflammatory MΦ (IMΦ), also termed TAM1 and tumor-supporting MΦ (TMΦ), also referred to as TAM2. Upon excessive inflammation, IMΦ can trigger cell death of parenchymal cells based on an disproportionate production of mediators such as the tumor necrosis factor (TNF). TMΦ supply tumors with growth factors and immunosuppressants, enabling tumor expansion and immune evasion.

Research of our group demonstrated M2 polarization *in vitro* by the two tripeptides RGD and GLF when coupled to gold nanorods [183]. However, the M2 polarization was not sufficient to treat acute liver inflammation. Unexpectedly, no therapeutic effects were observed at a dose analogue to the concentration used *in vitro*, the peptide-coupled particles even aggravated hepatic injury [184]. Subsequently, our research group put the focus to delivering anti-inflammatory drugs, particularly corticosteroids, to achieve M2-polarization [9] Using liposomal dexamethasone (Libode), we significantly reduced severity of Concanavalin A-induced autoimmune hepatitis, and even observed a reduced expression of fibrosis markers in the carbon tetrachloride (CCl_4)-based model of liver fibrosis [74]. Similarly, pathogenic inflammatory activation has similarly been achieved using small interfering RNA (siRNA) through a polymeric formulation [185].

In a very recent innovative study, macrophages were, together with a polarizing stimulus, encapsulated in an alginate matrix to be used as a production site for cytokines. These complexes were shown to inhibit the epithelial-to-mesenchymal (EMT) transition [186]. Repolarizing macrophages has been shown to work efficiently to induce tumor regression based on the delivery of an inducer for micro-RNA155 based on polypeptide nanovectors. These led to a 400-fold induction of the expression of miR155 in TAM and triggered them to express M1 and to repress M2 associated genes and proteins [187].

Ferumoxytol, an iron oxide-based drug which is normally used to treat anemia, reprograms M2 into M1-MΦ [188], which is desired to overcome the immunosuppressive activities of M2 in cancer. Yet, iron supplementation by feraheme can lead to side effects, particularly inflammation induced by iron overload. It thus remains a challenge to manipulate immune cells in a desired fashion. Alike the M1 polarization triggered by ferumoxtol, also Lipodex [9] and nanocarrier-coupled stavudine lead to inflammatory activation of MΦ [189], probably owed to an accumulation of the drug inside the cells. There are many strategies to combat lymphoid leukemia, *i.e.* by Rituximab and CAR-T cells, but there are few attempts to cure myeloid leukemia. One new drug for an improved therapy of acute myeloid leukemia is represented by CPX-351, a liposomal formulation which contains the two drugs cytarabine and daunorubicinin. CPX-351 efficiently targets and depletes myeloid cells, with a greater efficiency than the single administration of both drugs [19]. The drug is now approved by the FDA for treatment of acute myeloid leukemia (AML) [190]. The mechanism of action is hypothesized to be based on phagocytosis and subsequent elimination of the myeloid blasts.

Dendritic cells (DC) are the most efficient antigen-presenting cell and they are the cells which provide the selectivity to lymphocytes. Accordingly, targeting DC with appropriate (nano-)tools is a strong research direction [191]. Nano-sized vehicles enable improved vaccination processes since they can confer protection to biologically instable molecules, *i.e.* DNA or RNA. For instance, peptides that bear an antigen, DNA, or mRNA coding for antigens, or immunostimulatory oligonucleotides can be shielded off from the activities of proteases and endonucleases [191]. AuNP were demonstrated in own studies to to accumulate in the MHCII processing compartment of DC [183]. Specific modifications of nanocarriers can render the activation of the DC, and particularly conjugated peptides induce specific changes in the expression of DC maturation markers [183]. Nano-sized RNA-based lipoplexes, chaotic complexes of lipids and RNA, were demonstrated to enable vaccination against cancer [192].

In addition to targeting them in inflammatory diseases, neutrophils can also be targeted in the course of cancer treatment. However, studies on the potential of targeting them in cancer are limited. The scientists Acharyya and Massague have demonstrating that through interference with downstream targets of the MAPK cascade such as leukotriene biosynthesis, CXCR2, Anti-Bv8 and G-CSF antibodies, the outcome of tumor development can be influenced [193]. Recent studies revealed that combined targeting of neutrophils and macrophages, thus of tumor-associated neutrophils (TAN), and TAM precursors might open a novel avenue for cancer therapy [194].

CONCLUSIONS

Macrophages appear as a strong candidate for advanced cancer therapy, particularly in liver diseases and cancer. Various types of nanocarriers are predestined for them due to their phagocytic activities. The nanosystems have to be carefully designed by carefully choosing potential spacers, particle material, and putative ligands for targeting macrophage subpopulations. One major issue which may help to reduce long-term side effects is to enable biodegradability for nanoparticulates. In this regard, organic materials appear most feasible compared to inorganic, metal or metal-hybrid particles, which we have demonstrated to persist in different for weeks [5]. In the ideal case, nano-sized vectors should be degraded in the body after they fulfill their pharmaceutical action. Yet, not all types of organic particles are biodegradable, for instance, fullerenes or carbon nanotubes are not degradable [7].

Engagement of macrophages thus has to be done with caution, since there is a sensitive balance between the differentially polarized subsets which fulfill different functions. A putative overstimulation of M1 appears as a major goal in cancer therapy, could potentially result in inflammatory activation of macrophages what might lead to an unintended systemic inflammatory response as it is observed in in sepsis [195]. On the contrary, drug which aim to convert M1 in inflammatory disease into M2 cells might support cancer growth, since M2 were demonstrated to support cancer progression.

The route of administration represents a major issue for all nanomaterial-based drugs. From the perspective of patients, oral administration is preferred. However, this is nowadays mostly achieved by small molecule-based drugs given as tablets. Thus, a major drawback of nano-sized drugs is the necessity for parenteral administration such as subcutaneous or intravenous administration. In order to make oral administration possible, specific modulations of the drug formulation are required to enteral absorption and enterohepatic redistribution. Preclinical studies should therefore aim to establish an efficient strategy for targeting macrophages, which can subsequently be used to generate nanomedicines for oral delivery.

CONSENT FOR PUBLICATION

Not applicable.

CONFLICT OF INTEREST

The authors confirm that the contents of this chapter have no conflict of interest.

ACKNOWLEDGEMENTS

Declared none.

REFERENCES

[1]   Bartneck M. Immunomodulatory nanomedicine. Macromol Biosci. 2017; Published online on April 6.
[http://dx.doi.org/10.1002/mabi.201700021]

[2]   Nikoobakht B, Burda C, Braun M, Hun M, El-Sayed MA. The quenching of CdSe quantum dots photoluminescence by gold nanoparticles in solution. Photochem Photobiol 2002; 75(6): 591-7.
[http://dx.doi.org/10.1562/0031-8655(2002)075<0591:TQOCQD>2.0.CO;2] [PMID: 12081320]

[3]   Chen J, Saeki F, Wiley BJ, *et al.* Gold nanocages: bioconjugation and their potential use as optical imaging contrast agents. Nano Lett 2005; 5(3): 473-7.
[http://dx.doi.org/10.1021/nl047950t] [PMID: 15755097]

[4]   Krichevski O, Markovich G. Growth of colloidal gold nanostars and nanowires induced by palladium doping. Langmuir 2007; 23(3): 1496-9.
[http://dx.doi.org/10.1021/la062500x] [PMID: 17241079]

[5]   Bartneck M, Ritz T, Keul HA, *et al.* Peptide-functionalized gold nanorods increase liver injury in hepatitis. ACS Nano 2012; 6(10): 8767-77.
[http://dx.doi.org/10.1021/nn302502u] [PMID: 22994679]

[6]   Choi HS, Liu W, Misra P, *et al.* Renal clearance of quantum dots. Nat Biotechnol 2007; 25(10): 1165-70.
[http://dx.doi.org/10.1038/nbt1340] [PMID: 17891134]

[7]   Kümmerer K, Menz J, Schubert T, Thielemans W. Biodegradability of organic nanoparticles in the aqueous environment. Chemosphere 2011; 82(10): 1387-92.
[http://dx.doi.org/10.1016/j.chemosphere.2010.11.069] [PMID: 21195449]

[8]   Lammers T, Subr V, Ulbrich K, *et al.* HPMA-based polymer therapeutics improve the efficacy of surgery, of radiotherapy and of chemotherapy combinations. Nanomedicine (Lond) 2010; 5(10): 1501-23.
[http://dx.doi.org/10.2217/nnm.10.130] [PMID: 21143030]

[9]   Bartneck M, Peters FM, Warzecha KT, *et al.* Liposomal encapsulation of dexamethasone modulates cytotoxicity, inflammatory cytokine response, and migratory properties of primary human macrophages. Nanomedicine (Lond) 2014; 10(6): 1209-20.
[http://dx.doi.org/10.1016/j.nano.2014.02.011] [PMID: 24607939]

[10]   Jain TK, Reddy MK, Morales MA, Leslie-Pelecky DL, Labhasetwar V. Biodistribution, clearance, and biocompatibility of iron oxide magnetic nanoparticles in rats. Mol Pharm 2008; 5(2): 316-27.
[http://dx.doi.org/10.1021/mp7001285] [PMID: 18217714]

[11]   Pan Y, Neuss S, Leifert A, *et al.* Size-dependent cytotoxicity of gold nanoparticles. Small 2007; 3(11): 1941-9.
[http://dx.doi.org/10.1002/smll.200700378] [PMID: 17963284]

[12]   Shi H, Magaye R, Castranova V, Zhao J. Titanium dioxide nanoparticles: a review of current toxicological data. Part Fibre Toxicol 2013; 10: 15.
[http://dx.doi.org/10.1186/1743-8977-10-15] [PMID: 23587290]

[13]   Liu T, Li L, Fu C, Liu H, Chen D, Tang F. Pathological mechanisms of liver injury caused by continuous intraperitoneal injection of silica nanoparticles. Biomaterials 2012; 33(7): 2399-407.
[http://dx.doi.org/10.1016/j.biomaterials.2011.12.008] [PMID: 22182752]

[14]   Zelman WN, McLaughlin CP. Product lines in a complex marketplace: matching organizational strategy to buyer behavior. Health Care Manage Rev 1990; 15(2): 9-14.
[http://dx.doi.org/10.1097/00004010-199001520-00005] [PMID: 2351546]

[15]   Bartneck M, Keul HA, Singh S, *et al.* Rapid uptake of gold nanorods by primary human blood phagocytes and immunomodulatory effects of surface chemistry. ACS Nano 2010; 4(6): 3073-86.
[http://dx.doi.org/10.1021/nn100262h] [PMID: 20507158]

[16]   Bartneck M, Keul HA, Wambach M, *et al.* Effects of nanoparticle surface-coupled peptides, functional endgroups, and charge on intracellular distribution and functionality of human primary reticuloendothelial cells. Nanomedicine (Lond) 2012; 8(8): 1282-92.
[http://dx.doi.org/10.1016/j.nano.2012.02.012] [PMID: 22406188]

[17]   Bastús NG, Sánchez-Tilló E, Pujals S, *et al.* Homogeneous conjugation of peptides onto gold nanoparticles enhances macrophage response. ACS Nano 2009; 3(6): 1335-44.
[http://dx.doi.org/10.1021/nn8008273] [PMID: 19489561]

[18]   Havel H, Finch G, Strode P, *et al.* Nanomedicines: From bench to bedside and beyond. AAPS J 2016; 18(6): 1373-8.
[http://dx.doi.org/10.1208/s12248-016-9961-7] [PMID: 27480318]

[19]   Cortes JE, Goldberg SL, Feldman EJ, *et al.* Phase II, multicenter, randomized trial of CPX-351 (cytarabine:daunorubicin) liposome injection *versus* intensive salvage therapy in adults with first relapse AML. Cancer 2015; 121(2): 234-42.
[http://dx.doi.org/10.1002/cncr.28974] [PMID: 25223583]

[20]   Lancet JE, Cortes JE, Hogge DE, *et al.* Phase 2 trial of CPX-351, a fixed 5:1 molar ratio of cytarabine/daunorubicin, vs cytarabine/daunorubicin in older adults with untreated AML. Blood 2014; 123(21): 3239-46.
[http://dx.doi.org/10.1182/blood-2013-12-540971] [PMID: 24687088]

[21]   Bobo D, Robinson KJ, Islam J, Thurecht KJ, Corrie SR. Nanoparticle-based medicines: A review of FDA-approved materials and clinical trials to date. Pharm Res 2016; 33(10): 2373-87.
[http://dx.doi.org/10.1007/s11095-016-1958-5] [PMID: 27299311]

[22]   Caster JM, Patel AN, Zhang T, Wang A. Investigational nanomedicines in 2016: a review of nanotherapeutics currently undergoing clinical trials. Wiley Interdiscip Rev Nanomed Nanobiotechnol 2017; 9(1)
[http://dx.doi.org/10.1002/wnan.1416] [PMID: 27312983]

[23]   Havel HA. Where are the nanodrugs? An industry perspective on development of drug products containing nanomaterials. AAPS J 2016; 18(6): 1351-3.
[http://dx.doi.org/10.1208/s12248-016-9970-6] [PMID: 27520380]

[24]   Ventola CL. The nanomedicine revolution: part 1: emerging concepts. P & T : Form Manag. 2012; 37(9): 512-25.

[25]   Gao ZG, Lee DH, Kim DI, Bae YH. Doxorubicin loaded pH-sensitive micelle targeting acidic extracellular pH of human ovarian A2780 tumor in mice. J Drug Target 2005; 13(7): 391-7.
[http://dx.doi.org/10.1080/10611860500376741] [PMID: 16308207]

[26]   Koziara JM, Whisman TR, Tseng MT, Mumper RJ. *In-vivo* efficacy of novel paclitaxel nanoparticles in paclitaxel-resistant human colorectal tumors. J Control Rel Soc 2006; 112(3): 312-9.
[http://dx.doi.org/10.1016/j.jconrel.2006.03.001]

[27]   Lamprecht A, Benoit JP. Etoposide nanocarriers suppress glioma cell growth by intracellular drug delivery and simultaneous P-glycoprotein inhibition. J Control Rel Soc 2006; 112(2): 208-13.

[28]   Xu P, Van Kirk EA, Li S, *et al.* Highly stable core-surface-crosslinked nanoparticles as cisplatin carriers for cancer chemotherapy. Colloids Surf B Biointerfaces 2006; 48(1): 50-7.
[http://dx.doi.org/10.1016/j.colsurfb.2006.01.004] [PMID: 16497489]

[29]   Sutton D, Nasongkla N, Blanco E, Gao J. Functionalized micellar systems for cancer targeted drug delivery. Pharm Res 2007; 24(6): 1029-46.
[http://dx.doi.org/10.1007/s11095-006-9223-y] [PMID: 17385025]

[30]   Brigger I, Dubernet C, Couvreur P. Nanoparticles in cancer therapy and diagnosis. Adv Drug Deliv Rev 2002; 54(5): 631-51.
[http://dx.doi.org/10.1016/S0169-409X(02)00044-3] [PMID: 12204596]

[31]   Moghimi SM, Hunter AC, Murray JC. Long-circulating and target-specific nanoparticles: theory to practice. Pharmacol Rev 2001; 53(2): 283-318.
[PMID: 11356986]

[32]   Torchilin VP. Structure and design of polymeric surfactant-based drug delivery systems. J Control Rel Soc 2001;73(2-3):137-72.
[http://dx.doi.org/10.1016/S0168-3659(01)00299-1]

[33]   Kwon GS. Polymeric micelles for delivery of poorly water-soluble compounds. Crit Rev Ther Drug Carrier Syst 2003; 20(5): 357-403.
[http://dx.doi.org/10.1615/CritRevTherDrugCarrierSyst.v20.i5.20] [PMID: 14959789]

[34]   Lee RW, Shenoy DB, Sheel R. Micellar Nanoparticles: Applications for Topical and Passive Transdermal Drug Delivery Handbook of Non-invasive Drug Delivery Systems. Elsevier 2010; pp. 37-58.
[http://dx.doi.org/10.1016/B978-0-8155-2025-2.10002-2]

[35]   Ahn HK, Jung M, Sym SJ, *et al.* A phase II trial of Cremorphor EL-free paclitaxel (Genexol-PM) and gemcitabine in patients with advanced non-small cell lung cancer. Cancer Chemother Pharmacol 2014; 74(2): 277-82.
[http://dx.doi.org/10.1007/s00280-014-2498-5] [PMID: 24906423]

[36]   Kim DW, Kim SY, Kim HK, *et al.* Multicenter phase II trial of Genexol-PM, a novel Cremophor-free, polymeric micelle formulation of paclitaxel, with cisplatin in patients with advanced non-small-cell lung cancer. Ann Oncol 2007; 18(12): 2009-14.
[http://dx.doi.org/10.1093/annonc/mdm374] [PMID: 17785767]

[37]   Lee KS, Chung HC, Im SA, *et al.* Multicenter phase II trial of Genexol-PM, a Cremophor-free, polymeric micelle formulation of paclitaxel, in patients with metastatic breast cancer. Breast Cancer Res Treat 2008; 108(2): 241-50.
[http://dx.doi.org/10.1007/s10549-007-9591-y] [PMID: 17476588]

[38]   Kalomiraki M, Thermos K, Chaniotakis NA. Dendrimers as tunable vectors of drug delivery systems and biomedical and ocular applications. Int J Nanomed 2015; 11: 1-12.
[PMID: 26730187]

[39]   Kesharwani P, Jain K, Jain NK. Dendrimer as nanocarrier for drug delivery. Prog Polym Sci 2014; 39(2): 268-307.
[http://dx.doi.org/10.1016/j.progpolymsci.2013.07.005]

[40]   Biswas S, Torchilin VP. Dendrimers for siRNA Delivery. Pharmaceuticals (Basel) 2013; 6(2): 161-83.
[http://dx.doi.org/10.3390/ph6020161] [PMID: 24275946]

[41]   Somani S, Blatchford DR, Millington O, Stevenson ML, Dufes C. Transferrin-bearing polypropylenimine dendrimer for targeted gene delivery to the brain. J Control Rel Soc. 2014;188:78-86.
[http://dx.doi.org/10.1016/j.jconrel.2014.06.006]

[42]   Yang J, Zhang Q, Chang H, Cheng Y. Surface-engineered dendrimers in gene delivery. Chem Rev 2015; 115(11): 5274-300.
[http://dx.doi.org/10.1021/cr500542t] [PMID: 25944558]

[43]   Palmerston Mendes L, Pan J, Torchilin VP. Dendrimers as nanocarriers for nucleic acid and drug delivery in cancer therapy. Molecules 2017; 22(9): E1401.
[http://dx.doi.org/10.3390/molecules22091401] [PMID: 28832535]

[44]   Bielinska AU, Yen A, Wu HL, *et al.* Application of membrane-based dendrimer/DNA complexes for solid phase transfection *in vitro* and *in vivo*. Biomaterials 2000; 21(9): 877-87.
[http://dx.doi.org/10.1016/S0142-9612(99)00229-X] [PMID: 10735464]

[45]   Eichman JD, Bielinska AU, Kukowska-Latallo JF, Baker JR Jr. The use of PAMAM dendrimers in the efficient transfer of genetic material into cells. Pharm Sci Technol Today 2000; 3(7): 232-45.

[http://dx.doi.org/10.1016/S1461-5347(00)00273-X] [PMID: 10884679]

[46]   Kukowska-Latallo JF, Bielinska AU, Johnson J, Spindler R, Tomalia DA, Baker JR Jr. Efficient transfer of genetic material into mammalian cells using Starburst polyamidoamine dendrimers. Proc Natl Acad Sci USA 1996; 93(10): 4897-902.
[http://dx.doi.org/10.1073/pnas.93.10.4897] [PMID: 8643500]

[47]   Perez AP, Cosaka ML, Romero EL, Morilla MJ. Uptake and intracellular traffic of siRNA dendriplexes in glioblastoma cells and macrophages. Int J Nanomed 2011; 6: 2715-28.
[PMID: 22114502]

[48]   Perez AP, Romero EL, Morilla MJ. Ethylendiamine core PAMAM dendrimers/siRNA complexes as *in vitro* silencing agents. Int J Pharm 2009; 380(1-2): 189-200.
[http://dx.doi.org/10.1016/j.ijpharm.2009.06.035] [PMID: 19577619]

[49]   Choi JS, Lee EJ, Choi YH, Jeong YJ, Park JS. Poly(ethylene glycol)-block-poly(L-lysine) dendrimer: novel linear polymer/dendrimer block copolymer forming a spherical water-soluble polyionic complex with DNA. Bioconjug Chem 1999; 10(1): 62-5.
[http://dx.doi.org/10.1021/bc9800668] [PMID: 9893965]

[50]   Inoue Y, Kurihara R, Tsuchida A, Hasegawa M, Nagashima T, Mori T, *et al.* Efficient delivery of siRNA using dendritic poly(L-lysine) for loss-of-function analysis. J Control Rel Soc 2008;126(1):59-66.

[51]   Kaneshiro TL, Lu ZR. Targeted intracellular codelivery of chemotherapeutics and nucleic acid with a well-defined dendrimer-based nanoglobular carrier. Biomaterials 2009; 30(29): 5660-6.
[http://dx.doi.org/10.1016/j.biomaterials.2009.06.026] [PMID: 19595449]

[52]   Choudhary S, Gupta L, Rani S, Dave K, Gupta U. Impact of Dendrimers on Solubility of Hydrophobic Drug Molecules. Front Pharmacol 2017; 8: 261.
[http://dx.doi.org/10.3389/fphar.2017.00261] [PMID: 28559844]

[53]   Caminade A-M, Turrin C-O. Dendrimers for drug delivery. J Mater Chem B Mater Biol Med 2014; 2(26): 4055-66.
[http://dx.doi.org/10.1039/C4TB00171K] [PMID: 32261736]

[54]   Singh J, Jain K, Mehra NK, Jain NK. Dendrimers in anticancer drug delivery: mechanism of interaction of drug and dendrimers. Artif Cells Nanomed Biotechnol 2016; 44(7): 1626-34.
[http://dx.doi.org/10.3109/21691401.2015.1129625] [PMID: 26747336]

[55]   Bazak R, Houri M, El Achy S, Kamel S, Refaat T. Cancer active targeting by nanoparticles: a comprehensive review of literature. J Cancer Res Clin Oncol 2015; 141(5): 769-84.
[http://dx.doi.org/10.1007/s00432-014-1767-3] [PMID: 25005786]

[56]   Kulhari H, Pooja D, Shrivastava S, *et al.* Trastuzumab-grafted PAMAM dendrimers for the selective delivery of anticancer drugs to HER2-positive breast cancer. Sci Rep 2016; 6: 23179.
[http://dx.doi.org/10.1038/srep23179] [PMID: 27052896]

[57]   Chung A, Cui X, Audeh W, Giuliano A. Current status of anti-human epidermal growth factor receptor 2 therapies: predicting and overcoming herceptin resistance. Clin Breast Cancer 2013; 13(4): 223-32.
[http://dx.doi.org/10.1016/j.clbc.2013.04.001] [PMID: 23829888]

[58]   Borchard G, Flühmann B, Mühlebach S. Nanoparticle iron medicinal products - Requirements for approval of intended copies of non-biological complex drugs (NBCD) and the importance of clinical comparative studies. Regul Toxicol Pharmacol 2012; 64(2): 324-8.
[http://dx.doi.org/10.1016/j.yrtph.2012.08.009] [PMID: 22951348]

[59]   Danielson BG. Structure, chemistry, and pharmacokinetics of intravenous iron agents. J Am Soc Nephrol 2004; 15 (Suppl. 2): S93-8.
[PMID: 15585603]

[60]   Macdougall IC. Evolution of iv iron compounds over the last century. J Ren Care 2009; 35 (Suppl. 2):

8-13.
[http://dx.doi.org/10.1111/j.1755-6686.2009.00127.x] [PMID: 19891680]

[61]   Coyne DW, Auerbach M. Anemia management in chronic kidney disease: intravenous iron steps forward. Am J Hematol 2010; 85(5): 311-2.
[http://dx.doi.org/10.1002/ajh.21682] [PMID: 20232350]

[62]   Wolfram J, Zhu M, Yang Y, *et al.* Safety of Nanoparticles in Medicine. Curr Drug Targets 2015; 16(14): 1671-81.
[http://dx.doi.org/10.2174/1389450115666140804124808] [PMID: 26601723]

[63]   Libutti SK, Paciotti GF, Byrnes AA, *et al.* Phase I and pharmacokinetic studies of CYT-6091, a novel PEGylated colloidal gold-rhTNF nanomedicine. Clin Cancer Res 2010; 16(24): 6139-49.
[http://dx.doi.org/10.1158/1078-0432.CCR-10-0978] [PMID: 20876255]

[64]   Ali MR, Rahman MA, Wu Y, *et al.* Efficacy, long-term toxicity, and mechanistic studies of gold nanorods photothermal therapy of cancer in xenograft mice. Proc Natl Acad Sci USA 2017; 114(15): E3110-8.
[http://dx.doi.org/10.1073/pnas.1619302114] [PMID: 28356516]

[65]   Anselmo AC, Mitragotri S. Nanoparticles in the clinic. Bioeng Transl Med 2016; 1(1): 10-29.
[http://dx.doi.org/10.1002/btm2.10003] [PMID: 29313004]

[66]   Kharlamov AN, Tyurnina AE, Veselova VS, Kovtun OP, Shur VY, Gabinsky JL. Silica-gold nanoparticles for atheroprotective management of plaques: results of the NANOM-FIM trial. Nanoscale 2015; 7(17): 8003-15.
[http://dx.doi.org/10.1039/C5NR01050K] [PMID: 25864858]

[67]   Xu ZQ, Broza YY, Ionsecu R, *et al.* A nanomaterial-based breath test for distinguishing gastric cancer from benign gastric conditions. Br J Cancer 2013; 108(4): 941-50.
[http://dx.doi.org/10.1038/bjc.2013.44] [PMID: 23462808]

[68]   Müller RH, Maassen S, Weyhers H, Mehnert W. Phagocytic uptake and cytotoxicity of solid lipid nanoparticles (SLN) sterically stabilized with poloxamine 908 and poloxamer 407. J Drug Target 1996; 4(3): 161-70.
[http://dx.doi.org/10.3109/10611869609015973] [PMID: 8959488]

[69]   Bartneck M, Warzecha KT, Tacke F. Therapeutic targeting of liver inflammation and fibrosis by nanomedicine. Hepatobiliary Surg Nutr 2014; 3(6): 364-76.
[PMID: 25568860]

[70]   Lammers T, Aime S, Hennink WE, Storm G, Kiessling F. Theranostic nanomedicine. Acc Chem Res 2011; 44(10): 1029-38.
[http://dx.doi.org/10.1021/ar200019c] [PMID: 21545096]

[71]   van Essen M, Krenning EP, Kam BL, de Jong M, Valkema R, Kwekkeboom DJ. Peptide-receptor radionuclide therapy for endocrine tumors. Nat Rev Endocrinol 2009; 5(7): 382-93.
[http://dx.doi.org/10.1038/nrendo.2009.105] [PMID: 19488074]

[72]   Moog KE, Barz M, Bartneck M, *et al.* Polymeric Selectin Ligands Mimicking Complex Carbohydrates: From Selectin Binders to Modifiers of Macrophage Migration. Angew Chem Int Ed Engl 2017; 56(5): 1416-21.
[http://dx.doi.org/10.1002/anie.201610395] [PMID: 28005299]

[73]   Bartneck M, Schlößer CT, Barz M, *et al.* Immunomodulatory Therapy of Inflammatory Liver Disease Using Selectin-Binding Glycopolymers. ACS Nano 2017; 11(10): 9689-700.
[http://dx.doi.org/10.1021/acsnano.7b04630] [PMID: 28829572]

[74]   Bartneck M, Scheyda KM, Warzecha KT, *et al.* Fluorescent cell-traceable dexamethasone-loaded liposomes for the treatment of inflammatory liver diseases. Biomaterials 2015; 37: 367-82.
[http://dx.doi.org/10.1016/j.biomaterials.2014.10.030] [PMID: 25453965]

[75]   Gabizon A, Catane R, Uziely B, *et al.* Prolonged circulation time and enhanced accumulation in

malignant exudates of doxorubicin encapsulated in polyethylene-glycol coated liposomes. Cancer Res 1994; 54(4): 987-92.
[PMID: 8313389]

[76] Gabizon AA, Shmeeda H, Zalipsky S. Pros and cons of the liposome platform in cancer drug targeting. J Liposome Res 2006; 16(3): 175-83.
[http://dx.doi.org/10.1080/08982100600848769] [PMID: 16952872]

[77] Opazo F, Levy M, Byrom M, *et al*. Aptamers as potential tools for super-resolution microscopy. Nat Methods 2012; 9(10): 938-9.
[http://dx.doi.org/10.1038/nmeth.2179] [PMID: 23018995]

[78] Schulz C, Hecht J, Krüger-Genge A, Kratz K, Jung F, Lendlein A. Generating Aptamers Interacting with Polymeric Surfaces for Biofunctionalization. Macromol Biosci 2016; 16(12): 1776-91.
[http://dx.doi.org/10.1002/mabi.201600319] [PMID: 27689917]

[79] Szeitner Z, Lautner G, Nagy SK, Gyurcsányi RE, Mészáros T. A rational approach for generating cardiac troponin I selective Spiegelmers. Chem Commun (Camb) 2014; 50(51): 6801-4.
[http://dx.doi.org/10.1039/C4CC00447G] [PMID: 24836380]

[80] Barenholz Y. Doxil(R)--the first FDA-approved nano-drug: lessons learned. J Control Rel Soc 2012;160(2):117-34.

[81] Andral M. The physical alterations of the blood and animal fluids in disease: alterations of the blood in fever and inflammation. Prov Med Surg J (1840). 1841;2(47):419-21.

[82] Schneider LA, Korber A, Grabbe S, Dissemond J. Influence of pH on wound-healing: a new perspective for wound-therapy? Arch Dermatol Res 2007; 298(9): 413-20.
[http://dx.doi.org/10.1007/s00403-006-0713-x] [PMID: 17091276]

[83] Torchilin VP. Multifunctional, stimuli-sensitive nanoparticulate systems for drug delivery. Nat Rev Drug Discov 2014; 13(11): 813-27.
[http://dx.doi.org/10.1038/nrd4333] [PMID: 25287120]

[84] de la Rica R, Aili D, Stevens MM. Enzyme-responsive nanoparticles for drug release and diagnostics. Adv Drug Deliv Rev 2012; 64(11): 967-78.
[http://dx.doi.org/10.1016/j.addr.2012.01.002] [PMID: 22266127]

[85] Mura S, Nicolas J, Couvreur P. Stimuli-responsive nanocarriers for drug delivery. Nat Mater 2013; 12(11): 991-1003.
[http://dx.doi.org/10.1038/nmat3776] [PMID: 24150417]

[86] Topuz F, Bartneck M, Pan Y, Tacke F. One-Step Fabrication of Biocompatible Multifaceted Nanocomposite Gels and Nanolayers. Biomacromolecules 2017; 18(2): 386-97.
[http://dx.doi.org/10.1021/acs.biomac.6b01483] [PMID: 27977144]

[87] Varkouhi AK, Scholte M, Storm G, Haisma HJ. Endosomal escape pathways for delivery of biologicals. J Control Rel Soc 2011;151(3):220-8.
[http://dx.doi.org/10.1016/j.jconrel.2010.11.004]

[88] Hafez IM, Cullis PR. Tunable pH-sensitive liposomes. Methods Enzymol 2004; 387: 113-34.
[http://dx.doi.org/10.1016/S0076-6879(04)87007-1] [PMID: 15172160]

[89] Manning G, Whyte DB, Martinez R, Hunter T, Sudarsanam S. The protein kinase complement of the human genome. Science 2002; 298(5600): 1912-34.
[http://dx.doi.org/10.1126/science.1075762] [PMID: 12471243]

[90] Bai JPF, Melas IN, Hur J, Guo E. Advances in omics for informed pharmaceutical research and development in the era of systems medicine. Expert Opin Drug Discov 2018; 13(1): 1-4.
[http://dx.doi.org/10.1080/17460441.2018.1394839] [PMID: 29073782]

[91] Ferrari M. Cancer nanotechnology: opportunities and challenges. Nat Rev Cancer 2005; 5(3): 161-71.
[http://dx.doi.org/10.1038/nrc1566] [PMID: 15738981]

[92] Ritter JA, Ebner AD, Daniel KD, Stewart KL. Application of high gradient magnetic separation principles to magnetic drug targeting. J Magn Magn Mater 2004; 280(2): 184-201.
[http://dx.doi.org/10.1016/j.jmmm.2004.03.012]

[93] Cunningham CH, Arai T, Yang PC, McConnell MV, Pauly JM, Conolly SM. Positive contrast magnetic resonance imaging of cells labeled with magnetic nanoparticles. Magn Reson Med 2005; 53(5): 999-1005.
[http://dx.doi.org/10.1002/mrm.20477] [PMID: 15844142]

[94] Johannsen M, Gneveckow U, Eckelt L, *et al.* Clinical hyperthermia of prostate cancer using magnetic nanoparticles: presentation of a new interstitial technique. Int J Hyperthermia 2005; 21(7): 637-47.
[http://dx.doi.org/10.1080/02656730500158360] [PMID: 16304715]

[95] Jurgons R, Seliger C, Hilpert A, Trahms L, Odenbach S, Alexiou C. Drug loaded magnetic nanoparticles for cancer therapy. J Phys Condens Matter 2006; 18(38): S2893-902.
[http://dx.doi.org/10.1088/0953-8984/18/38/S24]

[96] Bogdanov A Jr, Wright SC, Marecos EM, *et al.* A long-circulating co-polymer in "passive targeting" to solid tumors. J Drug Target 1997; 4(5): 321-30.
[http://dx.doi.org/10.3109/10611869708995848] [PMID: 9169989]

[97] Bălăiţă L, Popa M. Polymer magnetic particles in biomedical applications. Revue Roumaine de Chimie 2009; 54:185-99.

[98] Rosengart AJ, Kaminski MD, Chen H, Caviness PL, Ebner AD, Ritter JA. Magnetizable implants and functionalized magnetic carriers: A novel approach for noninvasive yet targeted drug delivery. J Magn Magn Mater 2005; 293(1): 633-8.
[http://dx.doi.org/10.1016/j.jmmm.2005.01.087]

[99] Yellen BB, Forbes ZG, Halverson DS, *et al.* Targeted drug delivery to magnetic implants for therapeutic applications. J Magn Magn Mater 2005; 293(1): 647-54.
[http://dx.doi.org/10.1016/j.jmmm.2005.01.083]

[100] Liang K, Such GK, Johnston AP, *et al.* Endocytic pH-triggered degradation of nanoengineered multilayer capsules. Adv Mater 2014; 26(12): 1901-05.
[http://dx.doi.org/10.1002/adma.201305144]

[101] Ruan S, Cao X, Cun X, *et al.* Matrix metalloproteinase-sensitive size-shrinkable nanoparticles for deep tumor penetration and pH triggered doxorubicin release. Biomaterials 2015; 60: 100-10.
[http://dx.doi.org/10.1016/j.biomaterials.2015.05.006] [PMID: 25988725]

[102] Jochum FD, Theato P. Temperature- and light-responsive smart polymer materials. Chem Soc Rev 2013; 42(17): 7468-83.
[http://dx.doi.org/10.1039/C2CS35191A] [PMID: 22868906]

[103] Yang J, Shen D, Zhou L, Li W, Li X, Yao C, *et al.* Spatially Confined Fabrication of Core–Shell Gold Nanocages@Mesoporous Silica for Near-Infrared Controlled Photothermal Drug Release. Chem Mater 2013; 25(15): 3030-7.
[http://dx.doi.org/10.1021/cm401115b]

[104] Cheng YJ, Luo GF, Zhu JY, *et al.* Enzyme-induced and tumor-targeted drug delivery system based on multifunctional mesoporous silica nanoparticles. ACS Appl Mater Interfaces 2015; 7(17): 9078-87.
[http://dx.doi.org/10.1021/acsami.5b00752] [PMID: 25893819]

[105] Dzamukova MR, Naumenko EA, Lvov YM, Fakhrullin RF. Enzyme-activated intracellular drug delivery with tubule clay nanoformulation. Sci Rep 2015; 5: 10560.
[http://dx.doi.org/10.1038/srep10560] [PMID: 25976444]

[106] Hu Q, Katti PS, Gu Z. Enzyme-responsive nanomaterials for controlled drug delivery. Nanoscale 2014; 6(21): 12273-86.
[http://dx.doi.org/10.1039/C4NR04249B] [PMID: 25251024]

[107] Huang J, Shu Q, Wang L, Wu H, Wang AY, Mao H. Layer-by-layer assembled milk protein coated magnetic nanoparticle enabled oral drug delivery with high stability in stomach and enzyme-responsive release in small intestine. Biomaterials 2015; 39: 105-13.
[http://dx.doi.org/10.1016/j.biomaterials.2014.10.059] [PMID: 25477177]

[108] Ai X, Mu J, Xing B. Recent Advances of Light-Mediated Theranostics. Theranostics 2016; 6(13): 2439-57.
[http://dx.doi.org/10.7150/thno.16088] [PMID: 27877246]

[109] Bansal A, Zhang Y. Photocontrolled nanoparticle delivery systems for biomedical applications. Acc Chem Res 2014; 47(10): 3052-60.
[http://dx.doi.org/10.1021/ar500217w] [PMID: 25137555]

[110] Huang F, Liao WC, Sohn YS, Nechushtai R, Lu CH, Willner I. Light-Responsive and pH-Responsive DNA Microcapsules for Controlled Release of Loads. J Am Chem Soc 2016; 138(28): 8936-45.
[http://dx.doi.org/10.1021/jacs.6b04773] [PMID: 27309888]

[111] Karimi M, Sahandi Zangabad P, Baghaee-Ravari S, Ghazadeh M, Mirshekari H, Hamblin MR. Smart Nanostructures for Cargo Delivery: Uncaging and Activating by Light. J Am Chem Soc 2017; 139(13): 4584-610.
[http://dx.doi.org/10.1021/jacs.6b08313] [PMID: 28192672]

[112] Linsley CS, Wu BM. Recent advances in light-responsive on-demand drug-delivery systems. Ther Deliv 2017; 8(2): 89-107.
[http://dx.doi.org/10.4155/tde-2016-0060] [PMID: 28088880]

[113] Barhoumi A, Liu Q, Kohane DS. Ultraviolet light-mediated drug delivery: Principles, applications, and challenges. J Control Rel Soc 2015;219:31-42.

[114] Skirtach AG, Muñoz Javier A, Kreft O, et al. Laser-induced release of encapsulated materials inside living cells. Angew Chem Int Ed Engl 2006; 45(28): 4612-7.
[http://dx.doi.org/10.1002/anie.200504599] [PMID: 16791887]

[115] Yao C, Wang P, Li X, et al. Near-infrared-triggered azobenzene-liposome/upconversion nanoparticle hybrid vesicles for remotely controlled drug delivery to overcome cancer multidrug resistance. Adv Mat (Deerfield Beach, Fla). 2016;28(42):9341-8.

[116] Yi Q, Sukhorukov GB. UV light stimulated encapsulation and release by polyelectrolyte microcapsules. Adv Colloid Interface Sci 2014; 207: 280-9.
[http://dx.doi.org/10.1016/j.cis.2013.11.009] [PMID: 24370006]

[117] Yi Q, Sukhorukov GB. UV-induced disruption of microcapsules with azobenzene groups. Soft Matter 2014; 10(9): 1384-91.
[http://dx.doi.org/10.1039/C3SM51648B] [PMID: 24651273]

[118] Li X, Wang R, Zhang F, et al. Nd3+ sensitized up/down converting dual-mode nanomaterials for efficient in-vitro and in-vivo bioimaging excited at 800 nm. Sci Rep 2013; 3: 3536.
[http://dx.doi.org/10.1038/srep03536] [PMID: 24346622]

[119] Wang R, Li X, Zhou L, Zhang F. Epitaxial seeded growth of rare-earth nanocrystals with efficient 800 nm near-infrared to 1525 nm short-wavelength infrared downconversion photoluminescence for in-vivo bioimaging. Angew Chem Int Ed Engl 2014; 53(45): 12086-90.
[http://dx.doi.org/10.1002/anie.201407420] [PMID: 25196421]

[120] Wang R, Zhang F. NIR luminescent nanomaterials for biomedical imaging. J Mater Chem B Mater Biol Med 2014; 2(17): 2422-43.
[http://dx.doi.org/10.1039/c3tb21447h] [PMID: 32261412]

[121] Yan B, Boyer JC, Habault D, Branda NR, Zhao Y. Near infrared light triggered release of biomacromolecules from hydrogels loaded with upconversion nanoparticles. J Am Chem Soc 2012; 134(40): 16558-61.
[http://dx.doi.org/10.1021/ja308876j] [PMID: 23013429]

[122] Allen TM, Cullis PR. Liposomal drug delivery systems: from concept to clinical applications. Adv Drug Deliv Rev 2013; 65(1): 36-48.
       [http://dx.doi.org/10.1016/j.addr.2012.09.037] [PMID: 23036225]

[123] Papahadjopoulos D, Allen TM, Gabizon A, *et al.* Sterically stabilized liposomes: improvements in pharmacokinetics and antitumor therapeutic efficacy. Proc Natl Acad Sci USA 1991; 88(24): 11460-4.
       [http://dx.doi.org/10.1073/pnas.88.24.11460] [PMID: 1763060]

[124] Cabral H, Matsumoto Y, Mizuno K, *et al.* Accumulation of sub-100nm polymeric micelles in poorly permeable tumours depends on size. Nat Nanotechnol 2011; 6(12): 815-23.
       [http://dx.doi.org/10.1038/nnano.2011.166] [PMID: 22020122]

[125] Cheng R, Meng F, Deng C, Klok HA, Zhong Z. Dual and multi-stimuli responsive polymeric nanoparticles for programmed site-specific drug delivery. Biomaterials 2013; 34(14): 3647-57.
       [http://dx.doi.org/10.1016/j.biomaterials.2013.01.084] [PMID: 23415642]

[126] Stuart MA, Huck WT, Genzer J, *et al.* Emerging applications of stimuli-responsive polymer materials. Nat Mater 2010; 9(2): 101-13.
       [http://dx.doi.org/10.1038/nmat2614] [PMID: 20094081]

[127] Wu MX, Wang X, Yang YW. Polymer Nanoassembly as Delivery Systems and Anti-Bacterial Toolbox: From PGMAs to MSN@PGMAs. Chem Rec 2018; 18(1): 45-54.
       [http://dx.doi.org/10.1002/tcr.201700036] [PMID: 28675576]

[128] Gillies ER, Fréchet JM. Dendrimers and dendritic polymers in drug delivery. Drug Discov Today 2005; 10(1): 35-43.
       [http://dx.doi.org/10.1016/S1359-6446(04)03276-3] [PMID: 15676297]

[129] Lee JE, Lee N, Kim T, Kim J, Hyeon T. Multifunctional mesoporous silica nanocomposite nanoparticles for theranostic applications. Acc Chem Res 2011; 44(10): 893-902.
       [http://dx.doi.org/10.1021/ar2000259] [PMID: 21848274]

[130] Svenson S, Tomalia DA. Dendrimers in biomedical applications--reflections on the field. Adv Drug Deliv Rev 2005; 57(15): 2106-29.
       [http://dx.doi.org/10.1016/j.addr.2005.09.018] [PMID: 16305813]

[131] Abbaraju PL, Meka AK, Song H, *et al.* Asymmetric Silica Nanoparticles with Tunable Head-Tail Structures Enhance Hemocompatibility and Maturation of Immune Cells. J Am Chem Soc 2017; 139(18): 6321-8.
       [http://dx.doi.org/10.1021/jacs.6b12622] [PMID: 28440642]

[132] Chen C, Geng J, Pu F, Yang X, Ren J, Qu X. Polyvalent nucleic acid/mesoporous silica nanoparticle conjugates: dual stimuli-responsive vehicles for intracellular drug delivery. Angew Chem Int Ed Engl 2011; 50(4): 882-6.
       [http://dx.doi.org/10.1002/anie.201005471] [PMID: 21246683]

[133] Liu JN, Bu WB, Shi JL. Silica coated upconversion nanoparticles: a versatile platform for the development of efficient theranostics. Acc Chem Res 2015; 48(7): 1797-805.
       [http://dx.doi.org/10.1021/acs.accounts.5b00078] [PMID: 26057000]

[134] Shen D, Yang J, Li X, *et al.* Biphase stratification approach to three-dimensional dendritic biodegradable mesoporous silica nanospheres. Nano Lett 2014; 14(2): 923-32.
       [http://dx.doi.org/10.1021/nl404316v] [PMID: 24467566]

[135] Xiong L, Du X, Shi B, Bi J, Kleitz F, Qiao SZ. Tunable stellate mesoporous silica nanoparticles for intracellular drug delivery. J Mater Chem B Mater Biol Med 2015; 3(8): 1712-21.
       [http://dx.doi.org/10.1039/C4TB01601G] [PMID: 32262444]

[136] Xu C, Yu M, Noonan O, *et al.* Core-cone structured monodispersed mesoporous silica nanoparticles with ultra-large cavity for protein delivery. Small (Weinheim an der Bergstrasse, Germany). 2015;11(44):5949-55.
       [http://dx.doi.org/10.1002/smll.201501449]

[137] Zhao T, Nguyen NT, Xie Y, Sun X, Li Q, Li X. Inorganic nanocrystals functionalized mesoporous silica nanoparticles: fabrication and enhanced bio-applications. Front Chem 2017; 5: 118.
[http://dx.doi.org/10.3389/fchem.2017.00118] [PMID: 29326923]

[138] Deng K, Li C, Huang S, *et al.* Recent progress in near infrared light triggered photodynamic therapy. Small (Weinheim an der Bergstrasse, Germany). 2017;13(44).
[http://dx.doi.org/10.1002/smll.201702299]

[139] Li X, Zhang F, Zhao D. Lab on upconversion nanoparticles: optical properties and applications engineering *via* designed nanostructure. Chem Soc Rev 2015; 44(6): 1346-78.
[http://dx.doi.org/10.1039/C4CS00163J] [PMID: 25052250]

[140] Zhou B, Shi B, Jin D, Liu X. Controlling upconversion nanocrystals for emerging applications. Nat Nanotechnol 2015; 10(11): 924-36.
[http://dx.doi.org/10.1038/nnano.2015.251] [PMID: 26530022]

[141] Agasti SS, Chompoosor A, You CC, Ghosh P, Kim CK, Rotello VM. Photoregulated release of caged anticancer drugs from gold nanoparticles. J Am Chem Soc 2009; 131(16): 5728-9.
[http://dx.doi.org/10.1021/ja900591t] [PMID: 19351115]

[142] Chang Y, Cheng Y, Feng Y, *et al.* Resonance energy transfer-promoted photothermal and photodynamic performance of gold-copper sulfide yolk-shell nanoparticles for chemophototherapy of cancer. Nano Lett 2018; 18(2): 886-97.
[http://dx.doi.org/10.1021/acs.nanolett.7b04162] [PMID: 29323915]

[143] Deng X, Li K, Cai X, *et al.* A hollow-structured Cus@Cu₂ s@au nanohybrid: synergistically enhanced photothermal efficiency and photoswitchable targeting effect for cancer theranostics. Adv Mat (Deerfield Beach, Fla). 2017;29(36).

[144] Lin LS, Yang X, Zhou Z, *et al.* Yolk-shell nanostructure: an ideal architecture to achieve harmonious integration of magnetic-plasmonic hybrid theranostic platform. Adv Mat (Deerfield Beach, Fla). 2017;29(21).

[145] Liu S, Wang L, Lin M, *et al.* Cu(II)-Doped Polydopamine-Coated Gold Nanorods for Tumor Theranostics. ACS Appl Mater Interfaces 2017; 9(51): 44293-306.
[http://dx.doi.org/10.1021/acsami.7b13643] [PMID: 29235846]

[146] Zhou J, Jiang Y, Hou S, *et al.* Compact Plasmonic Blackbody for Cancer Theranosis in the Near-Infrared II Window. ACS Nano 2018; 12(3): 2643-51.
[http://dx.doi.org/10.1021/acsnano.7b08725] [PMID: 29438610]

[147] Li C, Yang D, Ma P, *et al.* Multifunctional upconversion mesoporous silica nanostructures for dual modal imaging and *in vivo* drug delivery. Small (Weinheim an der Bergstrasse, Germany). 2013;9(24):4150-9.
[http://dx.doi.org/10.1002/smll.201301093]

[148] Li Z, Zhang Y. Monodisperse silica-coated polyvinylpyrrolidone/NaYF(4) nanocrystals with multicolor upconversion fluorescence emission. Angew Chem Int Ed Engl 2006; 45(46): 7732-5.
[http://dx.doi.org/10.1002/anie.200602975] [PMID: 17089426]

[149] Liu J, Bu W, Zhang S, *et al.* Controlled synthesis of uniform and monodisperse upconversion core/mesoporous silica shell nanocomposites for bimodal imaging. Chemistry 2012; 18(8): 2335-41.
[http://dx.doi.org/10.1002/chem.201102599] [PMID: 22252972]

[150] Wu Z, Song N, Menz R, Pingali B, Yang YW, Zheng Y. Nanoparticles functionalized with supramolecular host-guest systems for nanomedicine and healthcare. Nanomedicine (Lond) 2015; 10(9): 1493-514.
[http://dx.doi.org/10.2217/nnm.15.1] [PMID: 25996121]

[151] Yang Y-W. Towards biocompatible nanovalves based on mesoporous silica nanoparticles. MedChemComm 2011; 2(11): 1033-49.
[http://dx.doi.org/10.1039/c1md00158b]

[152]   Sortino S. Photoactivated nanomaterials for biomedical release applications. J Mater Chem 2012; 22(2): 301-18.
[http://dx.doi.org/10.1039/C1JM13288A]

[153]   Yu H, Li J, Wu D, Qiu Z, Zhang Y. Chemistry and biological applications of photo-labile organic molecules. Chem Soc Rev 2010; 39(2): 464-73.
[http://dx.doi.org/10.1039/B901255A] [PMID: 20111771]

[154]   Pelliccioli AP, Wirz J. Photoremovable protecting groups: reaction mechanisms and applications. Photochem Photobiol Sci 2002; 1: 441–58.
[http://dx.doi.org/10.1039/b200777k]

[155]   Yang Y, Liu F, Liu X, Xing B. NIR light controlled photorelease of siRNA and its targeted intracellular delivery based on upconversion nanoparticles. Nanoscale 2013; 5(1): 231-8.
[http://dx.doi.org/10.1039/C2NR32835F] [PMID: 23154830]

[156]   Jayakumar MK, Idris NM, Zhang Y. Remote activation of biomolecules in deep tissues using near-infrared-to-UV upconversion nanotransducers. Proc Natl Acad Sci USA 2012; 109(22): 8483-8.
[http://dx.doi.org/10.1073/pnas.1114551109] [PMID: 22582171]

[157]   Lim LP, Lau NC, Garrett-Engele P, *et al.* Microarray analysis shows that some microRNAs downregulate large numbers of target mRNAs. Nature 2005; 433(7027): 769-73.
[http://dx.doi.org/10.1038/nature03315] [PMID: 15685193]

[158]   de Kerckhove M, Tanaka K, Umehara T, *et al.* Targeting *miR-223* in neutrophils enhances theclearance of *Staphylococcus aureus* in infectedwounds. EMBO Mol Med 2018; 10(10): e9024.
[http://dx.doi.org/10.15252/emmm.201809024] [PMID: 30171089]

[159]   Lam JK, Chow MY, Zhang Y, Leung SW. siRNA *versus* miRNA as therapeutics for gene silencing. Mol Ther Nucleic Acids 2015; 4: e252.
[http://dx.doi.org/10.1038/mtna.2015.23] [PMID: 26372022]

[160]   Roy S, Benz F, Luedde T, Roderburg C. The role of miRNAs in the regulation of inflammatory processes during hepatofibrogenesis. Hepatobiliary Surg Nutr 2015; 4(1): 24-33.
[PMID: 25713802]

[161]   Ledford H. Bankruptcy filing worries developers of nanoparticle cancer drugs. Nature 2016; 533(7603): 304-5.
[http://dx.doi.org/10.1038/533304a] [PMID: 27193658]

[162]   Rupaimoole R, Slack FJ. MicroRNA therapeutics: towards a new era for the management of cancer and other diseases. Nat Rev Drug Discov 2017; 16(3): 203-22.
[http://dx.doi.org/10.1038/nrd.2016.246] [PMID: 28209991]

[163]   Lv H, Zhang S, Wang B, Cui S, Yan J. Toxicity of cationic lipids and cationic polymers in gene delivery. J Control Rel Soc 2006;114(1):100-9.
[http://dx.doi.org/10.1016/j.jconrel.2006.04.014]

[164]   Hoy SM. Patisiran: First Global Approval. Drugs 2018; 78(15): 1625-31.
[http://dx.doi.org/10.1007/s40265-018-0983-6] [PMID: 30251172]

[165]   Jung G, Grosse-Hovest L, Krammer PH, Rammensee HG. Target cell-restricted triggering of the CD95 (APO-1/Fas) death receptor with bispecific antibody fragments. Cancer Res 2001; 61(5): 1846-8.
[PMID: 11280736]

[166]   Nalivaiko K, Hofmann M, Kober K, *et al.* A recombinant bispecific cd20xcd95 antibody with superior activity against normal and malignant B-cells. Mol Ther J Am Soc Gene Ther 2016;24(2):298-305.

[167]   Hoos A. Development of immuno-oncology drugs - from CTLA4 to PD1 to the next generations. Nat Rev Drug Discov 2016; 15(4): 235-47.
[http://dx.doi.org/10.1038/nrd.2015.35] [PMID: 26965203]

[168] Clement M, Pearson JA, Gras S, *et al.* Targeted suppression of autoreactive CD8⁺ T-cell activation using blocking anti-CD8 antibodies. Sci Rep 2016; 6: 35332.
[http://dx.doi.org/10.1038/srep35332] [PMID: 27748447]

[169] Panel OKs CAR T Therapy for Leukemia. Spreading colon cancer can bypass lymph nodes. Cancer Discov 2017; 7(9): 924.

[170] Jackson HJ, Rafiq S, Brentjens RJ. Driving CAR T-cells forward. Nat Rev Clin Oncol 2016; 13(6): 370-83.
[http://dx.doi.org/10.1038/nrclinonc.2016.36] [PMID: 27000958]

[171] Christensen AD, Skov S, Kvist PH, Haase C. Depletion of regulatory T cells in a hapten-induced inflammation model results in prolonged and increased inflammation driven by T cells. Clin Exp Immunol 2015; 179(3): 485-99.
[http://dx.doi.org/10.1111/cei.12466] [PMID: 25302741]

[172] Tyrsin D, Chuvpilo S, Matskevich A, *et al.* From TGN1412 to TAB08: the return of CD28 superagonist therapy to clinical development for the treatment of rheumatoid arthritis. Clin Exp Rheumatol 2016; 34(4) (Suppl. 98): 45-8.
[PMID: 27586803]

[173] Bilzer M, Roggel F, Gerbes AL. Role of Kupffer cells in host defense and liver disease. J Intern Assoc Stud 2006; 26(10): 1175-86.
[http://dx.doi.org/10.1111/j.1478-3231.2006.01342.x]

[174] Bartneck M, Keul HA, Zwadlo-Klarwasser G, Groll J. Phagocytosis independent extracellular nanoparticle clearance by human immune cells. Nano Lett 2010; 10(1): 59-63.
[http://dx.doi.org/10.1021/nl902830x] [PMID: 19994869]

[175] Bartneck M, Wang J. Therapeutic Targeting of Neutrophil Granulocytes in Inflammatory Liver Disease. Front Immunol 2019; 10: 2257.
[http://dx.doi.org/10.3389/fimmu.2019.02257] [PMID: 31616430]

[176] Xue J, Schmidt SV, Sander J, *et al.* Transcriptome-based network analysis reveals a spectrum model of human macrophage activation. Immunity 2014; 40(2): 274-88.
[http://dx.doi.org/10.1016/j.immuni.2014.01.006] [PMID: 24530056]

[177] Jenkins SJ, Ruckerl D, Cook PC, *et al.* Local macrophage proliferation, rather than recruitment from the blood, is a signature of TH2 inflammation. Science 2011; 332(6035): 1284-8.
[http://dx.doi.org/10.1126/science.1204351] [PMID: 21566158]

[178] Murray PJ, Allen JE, Biswas SK, *et al.* Macrophage activation and polarization: nomenclature and experimental guidelines. Immunity 2014; 41(1): 14-20.
[http://dx.doi.org/10.1016/j.immuni.2014.06.008] [PMID: 25035950]

[179] Bartneck M, Schrammen PL, Möckel D, *et al.* The CCR2⁺ Macrophage Subset Promotes Pathogenic Angiogenesis for Tumor Vascularization in Fibrotic Livers. Cell Mol Gastroenterol Hepatol 2019; 7(2): 371-90.
[http://dx.doi.org/10.1016/j.jcmgh.2018.10.007] [PMID: 30704985]

[180] Butt AQ, Mills KH. Immunosuppressive networks and checkpoints controlling antitumor immunity and their blockade in the development of cancer immunotherapeutics and vaccines. Oncogene 2014; 33(38): 4623-31.
[http://dx.doi.org/10.1038/onc.2013.432] [PMID: 24141774]

[181] Yona S, Kim KW, Wolf Y, *et al.* Fate mapping reveals origins and dynamics of monocytes and tissue macrophages under homeostasis. Immunity 2013; 38(1): 79-91.
[http://dx.doi.org/10.1016/j.immuni.2012.12.001] [PMID: 23273845]

[182] Bartneck M, Fech V, Ehling J, *et al.* Histidine-rich glycoprotein promotes macrophage activation and inflammation in chronic liver disease. Hepatology 2016; 63(4): 1310-24.
[http://dx.doi.org/10.1002/hep.28418] [PMID: 26699087]

[183] Bartneck M, Keul HA, Wambach M, *et al.* Effects of nanoparticle surface-coupled peptides, functional endgroups, and charge on intracellular distribution and functionality of human primary reticuloendothelial cells. Nanomedicine (Lond) 2012; 8(8): 1282-92.
[http://dx.doi.org/10.1016/j.nano.2012.02.012] [PMID: 22406188]

[184] Bartneck M. Current and rising concepts in immunotherapy: biopharmaceuticals *versus* nanomedicines. In: Bawa RJS, Webster JSt, Audette GF, Eds. Immune Aspects of Biopharmaceuticals and Nanomedicines. Singapore: Pan Stanford Publishing 2018.

[185] He C, Yin L, Tang C, Yin C. Multifunctional polymeric nanoparticles for oral delivery of TNF-α siRNA to macrophages. Biomaterials 2013; 34(11): 2843-54.
[http://dx.doi.org/10.1016/j.biomaterials.2013.01.033] [PMID: 23347838]

[186] Sola A, Saenz Del Burgo L, Ciriza J, *et al.* Microencapsulated macrophages releases conditioned medium able to prevent epithelial to mesenchymal transition. Drug Deliv 2018; 25(1): 91-101.
[http://dx.doi.org/10.1080/10717544.2017.1413449] [PMID: 29250977]

[187] Liu L, Yi H, He H, Pan H, Cai L, Ma Y. Tumor associated macrophage-targeted microRNA delivery with dual-responsive polypeptide nanovectors for anti-cancer therapy. Biomaterials 2017; 134: 166-79.
[http://dx.doi.org/10.1016/j.biomaterials.2017.04.043] [PMID: 28463694]

[188] Zanganeh S, Hutter G, Spitler R, *et al.* Iron oxide nanoparticles inhibit tumour growth by inducing pro-inflammatory macrophage polarization in tumour tissues. Nat Nanotechnol 2016; 11(11): 986-94.
[http://dx.doi.org/10.1038/nnano.2016.168] [PMID: 27668795]

[189] Zazo H, Colino CI, Warzecha KT, *et al.* Gold nanocarriers for macrophage-targeted therapy of human immunodeficiency virus. Macromol Biosci 2016; 17(3) : 1600359.
[PMID: 27748547]

[190] Nikanjam M, Capparelli EV, Lancet JE, Louie A, Schiller G. Persistent cytarabine and daunorubicin exposure after administration of novel liposomal formulation CPX-351: population pharmacokinetic assessment. Cancer Chemother Pharmacol 2018; 81(1): 171-8.
[http://dx.doi.org/10.1007/s00280-017-3484-5] [PMID: 29167924]

[191] Grabbe S, Landfester K, Schuppan D, Barz M, Zentel R. Nanoparticles and the immune system: challenges and opportunities. Nanomedicine (Lond) 2016; 11(20): 2621-4.
[http://dx.doi.org/10.2217/nnm-2016-0281] [PMID: 27649323]

[192] Grabbe S, Haas H, Diken M, Kranz LM, Langguth P, Sahin U. Translating nanoparticulate-personalized cancer vaccines into clinical applications: case study with RNA-lipoplexes for the treatment of melanoma. Nanomedicine (Lond) 2016; 11(20): 2723-34.
[http://dx.doi.org/10.2217/nnm-2016-0275] [PMID: 27700619]

[193] Acharyya S, Massague J. Arresting supporters: targeting neutrophils in metastasis. Cell Res 2016; 26(3): 273-4.
[http://dx.doi.org/10.1038/cr.2016.17] [PMID: 26823207]

[194] Kumar V, Donthireddy L, Marvel D, *et al.* Cancer-associated fibroblasts neutralize the anti-tumor effect of CSF1 receptor blockade by inducing PMN-MDSC infiltration of tumors. Cancer Cell 2017; 32(5): 654-68 e5.
[http://dx.doi.org/10.1016/j.ccell.2017.10.005]

[195] Schulte W, Bernhagen J, Bucala R. Cytokines in sepsis: potent immunoregulators and potential therapeutic targets--an updated view. Mediators Inflamm 2013; 2013: 165974.
[http://dx.doi.org/10.1155/2013/165974] [PMID: 23853427]

CHAPTER 4

Nanotheranostics in Gene Therapy

Beatriz B. Oliveira, Alexandra R. Fernandes and **Pedro V. Baptista**[*]

UCIBIO, Life Sciences Department, Faculdade de Ciências e Tecnologia, Campus de Caparica, 2829-516 Caparica, Portugal

Abstract: The continuous advances in molecular genetics have prompt for a wealth of tools capable to modulate genome and the corresponding gene expression. These innovative technologies have broadened the range of possibilities for gene therapy, either to decrease expression of malignant genes and mutations or edition of genomes for correction of errors. These strategies rely on the delivery of therapeutic nucleic acids to cells and tissues that must overcome several biological barriers. Indeed, a key element for the success of any gene therapy formulation is the carrier agent capable to deliver the therapeutic nucleic acid moieties to a specific target and promote efficient cellular uptake, while preventing deleterious off-target effects and degradation by endogenous nucleases. The initial vectorization strategies proved to be rather immunogenic, limited in the amount of genetic material that can be packed and raised severe toxicity concerns. Nowadays, a new generation of nanotechnology-based gene delivery systems are making an impact on the way we use therapeutic nucleic acids. These nanovectorization platforms have been developed so as to show low immunogenicity, low toxicity, ease of assembly and scale-up with higher loading capacity. Some of these nanoscale systems have also allowed for controlled release system and for the simultaneous capability of monitorization of effect – nanotheranostics. Herein, we provide a review on the variety of gene delivery vectors and platforms at the nanoscale.

Keywords: Cancer, Gene therapy, Nanomedicine, Nanotheranostics, RNAi.

1. GENE DELIVERY FOR CANCER THERAPY

In 2016, cancer accounted for more than 16% of the all deaths worldwide [1], with surgery, radiotherapy, chemotherapy, immune or hormone therapy being the standard procedures to manage tumors caused by gene mutations, deficiency or overexpression. Despite their valuable application, 95% of all new therapeutics show poor pharmacokinetics and/or biopharmaceutical properties and side effects

---

[*] **Corresponding author Pedro V. Baptista:** UCIBIO, Department Life Sciences, Faculdade de Ciências e Tecnologia, Universidade NOVA de Lisboa, 2829-516 Caparica, Portugal; Tel: +351 21 2948530; E-mail: pmvb@fct.unl.pt

Yusuf Tutar (Ed.)

that may limit their clinical application [2]. Hence, the ultimate challenge is to develop effective, nontoxic, non-immunogenic, noncarcinogenic vectors to deliver nucleic acids and/or drugs into cells, to achieve selective delivery of therapeutics to target areas in the body, minimizing their side effects and increasing their efficiency [3, 4]. Hence, the approval of novel gene/drug delivery platforms for cancer management is now a critical need [5].

Broadly, gene therapy consists in the manipulation of cells genetic information at the nucleic acid level, for the correction or modification of defective and/or missing gene sequences, so as to cure inherited and/or acquired diseases [3, 6]. In the last decades, with the discovery of novel small RNA molecules and their important role in the regulation of cell function, RNA has become both the target and the effector of a range of novel therapeutics [7]. RNA therapeutics refers to the use of oligonucleotides (DNA or RNA) to target RNA molecules for therapeutic needs. Currently, there are two major approaches in RNA therapeutics that have already been tested in the clinics: double-stranded RNA-mediated interference (RNAi) and antisense oligonucleotides (ASO) [8]. ASOs act *via* bind to their nucleic acid target by Watson-Crick base paring, inhibiting or altering the gene expression through steric hindrance, initiation of target degradation, splicing alterations or other events. RNAi operates *via* sequence specific and post-transcriptional modulation, preventing translation into proteins, through the activation of ribonucleases and other enzyme complexes that co-ordinately degrade the targeted RNA molecules [9]. RNAi therapeutics can be achieved though the design of specific RNAi regulators, such as microRNAs (miRNAs) mimics and small interfering RNAs (siRNAs). Antagomirs are novel synthetic single-stranded miRNA analogues with 21-23 nucleotides of range, that have been recently developed specifically for miRNA silencing. The use of this native mechanism for therapeutic and diagnostic purposes can be achieved by exogenous delivery of synthetic RNAi molecules. However, due to their negative charge and relatively large size, RNAi molecules are less likely to readily cross the biological barriers. Therefore, carrier systems and chemical modifications are needed, to protect the RNAi molecules, allowing an effective systemic delivery to the site of action. Importantly, carrier systems provide a simplified manner of cell penetration maintaining the functionality of RNAi molecules [10, 11].

More recently, a new class of nucleic acid-based therapeutics have been proposed for application in a wide range of diseases - precision genome editing using the clustered regularly interspaced short palindromic repeats (CRISPR)-CRISPR associated 9 (Cas9) technology [12]. Indeed, with Cas9, a RNA-guided endonuclease, it is possible to engineer DNA double strand breaks (DSB) at specific *loci*, thus editing the genome at precise locations. Several applications of CRISPR technology for gene inactivation and genome editing have been reported in humans [13]. This CRISPR-Cas9 strategy was preceded by other editing schemes that rely on altering endogenous molecular machinery to edit target regions of genomic DNA, such as zinc fingers nucleases (ZFN, that fuse the capability of zinc fingers domains to recognized DNA target sequences and nuclease activity), transcription activator-like effector nucleases (TALEN, that fuse a TAL effector DNA-binding domain to a DNA nuclease domain), among others [14 - 16]. Still, these pioneering concepts have had a small impact beyond preliminary studies as proof-of-concept and, as such, not yet translated to the clinical setting.

Having all these new technologies available is of cumbersome relevance, but a key element is crucial for the success of any gene therapy formulation: the carrier agent. Primary challenges are the delivery of the therapeutic nucleic acid moieties to a specific target and the efficient cellular uptake [17]. First generation of carriers were viral vectors, capable to mediate gene transfer with high efficiency and provide for long-term gene expression. However, they are rather immunogenic, show limitations in the amount of genetic material that can be packed and have raised severe toxicity concerns [18]. These drawbacks have prompted for development of non-viral alternatives for gene delivery showing low immunogenicity, low toxicity, ease of assembly and scale-up, and higher loading capacity [19]. The critical parameters of the carrier include size, shape, ligand functionalization and surface charge, that dictate the level of protection of the therapeutic nucleic acid against degradation and the pathway of cell uptake [18]. Moreover, a successful approach should include a controlled release system. This paved the way for the development and optimization of nanotechnology-based delivery of gene therapy. Herein, we shall provide a review on the diversity of gene delivery vectors and platforms at nanoscale and their applications.

2. NANOTECHNOLOGY IN GENE DELIVERY

Nanotechnology (and/or nanoscale) systems show unique properties that have been explores towards the development of conceptual therapeutic and diagnostic platforms, including *in vivo* imaging of drug delivery [20]. Some of these concepts have been further developed and several clinical trials demonstrate the powerful impact of nanotechnology-based systems in molecular therapeutics. Perhaps, the strongest impact has been felt in the field of cancer therapeutics, where nanomedicine has been showing great promise for controlled and targeted delivery of drugs and molecular actuators for gene therapy. Understanding the molecular causes of cancer had a major contribute on the design of targeted gene delivery [21].

2.1. Considering the Biological Barriers

Regardless of the type of vector, material and targeting method, the success of transfection is mostly dictated by the ability of the carrier to overcome the biological barriers to gene delivery. As mentioned above, non-viral vectors have more difficulties in gene delivery than their viral counterparts. This inefficiency mainly results from incapacity of gene complexes to surpass the numerous obstacles encountered from the site of administration to cell nucleus, and from there again to the cytoplasm where the transgenes are translated into proteins.

Biological barriers are generally divided into extracellular and intracellular barriers (Fig. **1**). The former includes: 1) nanoconjugate's stability in the body; 2) blood components and opsonization and 3) endothelial barriers (*i.e.* blood-brain barrier, vitreous humor, respiratory mucus). Most of these extracellular barriers can influence biodistribution of the administered vectors which in turn influences their bioavailability in the target cells [22]. For instance, positively charged NPs tend to be absorbed by polyanionic proteins, like proteoglycans, that are usually covalently cross-linked with serum albumin and other extracellular proteins large aggregates and are rapidly cleared by phagocyte system [23]. On the other hand, intracellular barriers include: 1) cellular binding; 2) cellular uptake; 3) endosomal/lysosomal escape and 4) potential nuclear entry.

As the nanoconjugate encounters each one of these barriers, the probability of a successful gene delivery drops significantly which correlates more to the type of carrier than to any other parameter. For instance, the internalization of lipoplexes occurs *via* endocytosis. Some of the endocytic pathways include caveolae and clathrin-independent, caveolae-mediated and micropinocytosis. Lipoplex diameter determines the pathway of entry, which correlates directly to transfection efficiency [24, 25]. Such situation was demonstrated in a gene transfection efficiency study of lipid-based carrier agents of DOTAP and DOPE, on Chinese hamster ovary cells [26].

The effective delivery of the therapeutic nucleic acid payload to the desired cell must consider the type of targeting approach provided by the nanoplatform, either active or passive. Passive targeting relies on the Enhanced Permeability and Retention (EPR) effect, in which nanocarriers extravasate preferentially at the tumor site due to the leaky microvasculature caused by increased angiogenesis and inflammation, the presence of cytokines and other vasoactive factors that enhance permeability [27]. Active targeting relies on the modification of the vector's surface with specific ligands (*e.g.* antibodies, peptides, sugars, aptamers, *etc.*) that are recognized by target cells/tissues and enhance adsorption and binding, resulting in selective cell uptake [28].

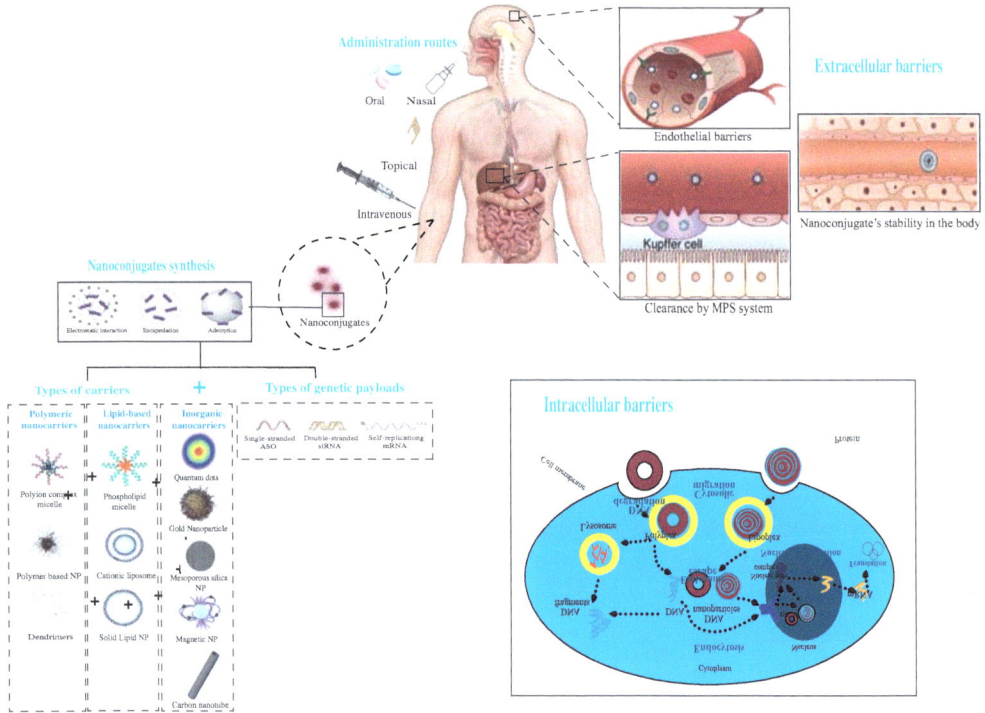

Fig. (1). Nanoconjugates can enter the body through nasal, oral, topical and intravenous administration. The most important role of nanoconjugates is to protect and deliver the genetic payloads to their target sites. There are various types of non-viral carriers, each one with its own advantages and drawbacks. Additionally, the genetic payloads also varie accordingly to the type of therapeutic target. The nanoconjugate combines the carrier agent with the genetic payload, that can be performed by electrostatic interaction, encapsulation or adsorption. From the administration site through the target site the nanoconjugate encounters innumerous obstacles like the biological barriers. The ability of the nanoconjugate to surpass these biological barriers is the key point to the success of the therapy. Biological barriers can be divided in two types: extracellular and intracellular. The extracellular barriers include: 1) Nanoconjugate's stability in the body; 2) The endothelial barriers; and 3) the clearance by the Mononuclear Phagocyte System (MPS). The intracellular barriers include: 1) The internalization of the nanoconjugates after binding to the cell membrane not occur; 2) Following endocytosis, a portion of the genetic payload could be degraded by the acidic late endosomes and lysosomes; 3) Endosomal escape; 4) After successful endosomal escape, the genetic payload could be further degraded by cytoplasmic DNAse (if the genetic payload is DNA) during the cytosolic migration to the cell nucleus; 5) The portion of the genetic payload that was able to reach the nucleus may be unable to induce transcription; and 6) some of the exported mRNA could be unable of translation into a functional transgenic protein.

The ability of nanoconjugates to alter gene expression depends not only on their local concentration, but also on the presence of extracellular matrix (ECM) proteins and substrate surface chemistry [18]. Additional PEG coating prevents unspecific interactions between the gene-loaded NP and plasma components. It also improves solubility, decreases the tendency of aggregation and increases the circulation time in the body by delaying opsonization and recognition followed by removal from circulation by the reticuloendothelial system (RES) [29].

Moreover, therapeutic nucleic acids may also encounter many enzymes with the potential to degrade them straightaway, like the DNase and RNases, serum proteases, and pH variations. To avoid degradation of genetic material and ensure high transfection efficiency, the nanocarrier must protect the therapeutic gene from the cellular environment, by encapsulation or electrostatic binding [30]. These issues can usually be solved by conjugation of the genetic material with a variety of cationic substrates, such as liposomes and polymers [31].

2.2. Gene Delivery Systems and Applications

A wide variety of organic and inorganic materials can be used for assembling nanoplatforms for gene delivery, such as lipids (liposomes, nanoemulsions and solid-liquid nanoparticles), polymers (biodegradable and nonbiodegradable), graphene, carbon nanotubes (CNTs), nanospheres, mesoporous nanoparticles (NPs) and other types of inorganic NPs, amphiphilic molecules, dendrimers, metals and semiconductor nanocrystals (quantum dots) [32]. The choice of the vector's material is mainly dictated by the desired application, type of cargo, route of administration and safety profile. Taking advantage of the synergistic effects among all these materials is the key to the development of better nanomaterials for gene delivery applications. The main applications, advantages and disadvantages of each of these systems are described in Table **1**. Still, when we consider the long track record and the clinical translation, currently, liposomes and polymer micro/nanoparticles are two of the most accessed systems for gene and drug delivery [33].

When considering cancer, which may be confined to specific locations in the body or may be disseminated in small foci, directing these carriers selectively to the tumor cells is of critical relevance to ensure efficacy. As such, considering that, due to the nanoscale dimensions of these carriers, will profit from EPR to passively accumulate to the tumor, active targeting plays a critical role in directing the delivery of the gene therapeutics to the relevant target. Besides the physic-chemical characteristics that provide the passive targeting, these nanovectors may be coupled/combined to active targeting moieties for selective uptake by the malignant tissues and cells, thus enhancing therapeutic efficacy while decreasing deleterious side effects to healthy tissues.

Table 1. Types of nanocarriers for gene delivery in cancer.

Nanocarrier	Description	Advantages	Disadvantages	Ref.
Cationic liposomes	• Amphiphilic molecules with positive charge • Conjugation of a positive and a neutral lipid • Attract the negatively charged phosphate groups of DNA molecule forming a lipoplex • Most used gene delivery vehicle	• Self-assembly interaction with DNA • Approved for pharmaceutical applications in humans • High chemical stability and biodegradability • Enhanced target specificity, cell uptake and trafficking • Cell interaction through electrostatic interactions • Can be coupled to pH-sensitive controlled release system that enhances endosomal escape	• High positive charge density at the NPs surface results in reduced gene transfection and higher cytotoxicity	[35, 57-65]
Solid lipid NPs (SLNs)	• High melting point lipids that act like a solid core, covered by surfactants • Cationic SLNs, such as CTAB, bind to DNA *via* electrostatic interactions	• Self-assembly interaction with DNA • Mostly recognized as safe • Approved for pharmaceutical applications in humans • Lower toxicity, smaller diameter, higher transfection efficiency *in vitro*, than liposomes equivalents • High stability which enables industrial production	• Provide for low transient expression levels • Toxicity issues	[36, 37, 40, 41]

(Table 1) cont.....

Nanocarrier	Description	Advantages	Disadvantages	Ref.
Polymer-based NPs	• Cationic polymers are the second most used group of non-viral vectors in gene delivery applications • Condense and neutralize the genetic material to form nanosized complexes, known as polyplexes	• Self-assembly interaction with DNA • Smaller size, narrow distribution, higher protection against nucleases and higher control of physical properties, when compared to lipid-based systems • Enhanced cell binding and transfection efficiency • Controlled release kinetics • Adjustable charge distribution through copolymerization with different polymers	• High cytotoxicity (optimal polymer size needs to balance transfection efficiency with cytotoxicity) • High immunogenicity • DNA degradation upon gene delivery • Excessive fast or slow release kinetics of the encapsulated gene	[52, 66 – 73]
Polyion Complex (PIC) micelle	• PLL-PEG copolymer, in which PLL segments and pDNA form a hydrophobic core, through hydrostatic interactions, and PEG acts as a hydrophilic coating layer	• Colloidal stability in protein aqueous media, when compared with conventional lipoplex and polyplex systems • Novel PIC micelles include stimuli sensitivity	• Several factors need to be optimized during the formulation of PIC micelles • Need to overcome issues with toxicity, stability, cellular uptake, endosomal escape and nuclei delivery for nucleic acids.	[74 – 76]
Peptide-based NPs	• Peptide/DNA complexes formed by electrostatic interactions between negatively charged DNA and short peptides containing positively charged amino acids, such as histidine, lysine and arginine	• Prevention of DNA degradation by nucleases • Prolonged circulation time. • The positive charge exhibited by peptide/DNA complexes facilitates the interaction with cell membranes and internalization into the cell • Enables endosomal/ lysosomal escape	• Fabrication of peptide nanomaterials for biomedical applications in a controllable and predictive way is not possible yet, due to difficulties in the manipulation of non-covalent interactions.	[77, 78]

(Table 1) cont.....

Nanocarrier	Description	Advantages	Disadvantages	Ref.
Graphene-based nanomaterials	• Graphene oxide (GO) nanostructures • Surface modification with cationic polymers prevents electrostatic repulsion between both negatively charged naked surface of graphene-based NPs and phosphate backbone of DNA molecule	• Large surface area, easy functionalization process and excellent electrical and thermal conductivities • Enables a wide range of surface modifications	• Must be coated with cationic polymers such as PEI to avoid its interaction with other biomolecules	[79, 80]
Quantum dots (QDs)	• Luminescent semiconductor nanocrystals • Synthetized from binary combinations of semiconductor materials such as ZnS, CdS, CdTe, InP, PbTe. • The most widely used are made of CdSe/ZnS and CdTe/ZnS	• Powerful visualization tool for biolabeling and bioimaging applications, such as theranostic systems. • New generation of probes with combined functionalities of labeling and gene/drug delivery • NPs could be successfully delivered to their target sites with simultaneously monitorization of their fluorescence intensity in real time	• Cytotoxicity • Requires conjugation with other nanomaterials for effective gene delivery	[81 – 84]
Magnetic NPs (MNPs)	• Composed by a magnetic core, an organic coating and multiple functional molecules on their surface • Most commonly used coating agents are cationic polymers such as chitosan, PEI and PAMAM so that negatively charged nucleic acids can absorb or condense.	• In addition to their protection effect, coating polymers also play an important role in the enhancement of superparamagnetic iron oxide NPs (SPIONs) pharmacokinetics and endosomal escape • Allow tracking through MRI and have gained much consideration as gene delivery and theranostic systems	• Have to be covered with the proper materials, in order to both isolate them from the biological environment (avoiding contact with blood-proteins and phagocytosis associated receptors) and protection against acid or base corrosion and oxidation	[85, 86]

(Table 1) cont.....

Nanocarrier	Description	Advantages	Disadvantages	Ref.
Gold NPs (AuNPs)	• Composed by a gold core and the surface can be modified/ functionalized with a great variety of compounds. • AuNPs can be prepared by the reduction of gold salts in the presence of appropriate stabilizing agents that prevent particle agglomeration.	• The gold core is essentially inert and nontoxic. • Easy synthesis. • Ready functionalization allows a great versatility. • Great capacity of encapsulate payloads with different sizes, such as small drug molecules and large biomolecules like proteins, DNA or RNA. • Photophysical properties could trigger drug/gene delivery at remote sites.	• The original capping agents of some AuNPs such as gold nanorods may be cytotoxic. • Despite the nontoxicity of the gold core some toxicity may be specific to some ligands.	[87, 88]

2.3. Targeting Strategies

In passive targeting, macromolecules including nanoparticles and other carrier systems accumulate preferentially in the neoplastic tissues as a result of the EPR effect first described by Maeda and Matsumura [34, 35]. The distinctive characteristics of the tumor microenvironment facilitates the deposition of nanoconjugates at the tumor site. These characteristics include leaky vasculature and impaired lymphatic drainage, which normally are not present in the healthy tissues. The lack of the smooth muscle cells, which is essential for mediating a vasogenic response, in tumor tissue is responsible for a state of permanent vasodilatation and non-responsiveness to physiological stimuli regulating the blood flow [36]. So, these aberrant neoplastic vessels result in abnormal transport dynamics of fluid and solutes across the tumor vessels, which may be responsible for accentuating the EPR phenomenon in this type of tissues and consequently allows its exploitation for therapeutic applications [37]. In fact, studies in animal models have shown that the EPR effect can lead to a 50-fold accumulation in tumors comparing with healthy tissues [38].

Various sizes, compositions and types of nanoparticles had their tumor interaction described as EPR effect, including micelles [39], liposomes [40], polymeric nanoparticles [41] and nanosized materials up to 400nm in diameter. However, solely relying on the EPR effect might not be enough for theranostics success, due to tumor heterogenicity, the inability of the NP to reach central regions of the tumor [42], and the fact that not all types of tumor allow accumulation *via* EPR, including gastric and pancreatic cancers [43].

The active targeting strategy depends on the affinity ligands that will directly bind the nanoparticles to overexpressed receptors on tumor surfaces [44]. This can be achieved by decorating the surface of the NP with targeting elements including antibodies, peptide fragments and nucleic acid ligands [45].

Antibodies

The only class of targeting ligands that are currently clinically available are antibodies [46]. They have consistently shown an increase in cellular uptake comparing to non-targeted nanoparticles [47]. However, large monoclonal antibodies have downsides, which include their large size that can affect the stability and diameter of the NPs, the reproducibility of the assays and raise immunogenicity concerns [48]. There are many proteins available that will bind to overexpressed membrane receptors and can be used to target cancer cells and evade normal cells [*e.g.* anti-epidermal growth factor receptor (anti-EGFR)] [49]. One example regards the use of anti-EGFR antibody conjugated gold nanoparticles as a theranostic system. The efficient conversion of the light absorbed by the plasmonic gold nanoparticles in heat and the their easy bioconjugation suggests that the conjugate propose by El-Sayed *et al.* could be used as selective photothermal agents in molecular cancer cell targeting [50].

Peptides

Peptides used for targeting have 2 to 50 amino acids in their constitution [51]. There are a number of peptide receptors overexpressed in tumor cells, such as luteinizing hormone-releasing hormone (LHRH), bombesin receptor, and somatostatin. Moreover, peptides can also be used to target integrins that are normally overexpressed in tumor neo-vasculature [52]. The advantages of using peptides as targeting ligands include their small size, high stability, high binding affinity, ease of synthesis and clearance [53]. Short peptide fragments possess advantages over larger antibody fragments, because they are intrinsically smaller, less immunogenic, have more stability and are easier to produce. Although, small peptides have less affinity than antibodies, this issue is usually surpassed by increasing the number of targeting peptides on the NPs surface which leads to an increase in avidity [54]. In fact, Pedrosa *et al.* presents an example of targeting tumor angiogenesis with peptide functionalized gold nanoparticles. In this study is proposed the combination of green laser irradiation with administration of AuNPs functionalized with an anti-angiogenic peptide for focalized phototherapy towards blockade of neovascularization *in vivo* [55].

Small Molecules

Small molecules are used as targeting elements due to their low molecular weight, ease of conjugation to NPs through a number of techniques, low immunogenic effects, lack of degradation and low production costs. Moreover, their small size allows NPs to be packed with a high number of molecules, thus increasing the probability of targeting success. Due to the overexpression of folic acid receptor (FR) in many types of cancer cells including brain, breast, lung, bone, head and neck, folic acid is one the most researched small molecule for targeting applications [56]. Its numerous benefits include non-immunogenicity [57]. The various platforms offer a tremendous potential for nanomedicine improvement, since they allow the enhancement of treatment options, earlier detection and monitorization of disease phase, which truly leads to precision medicine.

3. NANOTHERANOSTICS CONCEPTS FOR GENE DELIVERY

Theranostics refers to the combination of therapy and diagnostic into a single multifunctional formulation [89]. In fact, a theranostic system could be interpreted as the combination of therapeutic compounds and diagnostic agents that promises better prognostics, fewer side effects and improved treatments, even for fatal diseases such as cancer [90]. Nanotheranostics applies and develops nanomedicine strategies, using multiple nanocarriers (*i.e.,* polymer conjugates, micelles, dendrimers, liposomes, metal and inorganic nanoparticles, carbon nanotubes and nanoparticles of biodegradable polymers) for sustained, controlled and targeted co-delivery of diagnostic and therapeutic agents [91]. To achieve this multifunctionality on a theranostic formulation, four components are usually required: 1) nanoparticle or other delivery vehicle; 2) diagnostic/imaging domain; 3) targeting ligand and 4) therapeutic agent. Still, several considerations should also be made in the design of the theranostic formulation, such as the type of nanoparticle (*i.e.,* polymers, liposomes, dendrimers, polymeric micelles), size, shape, charge and surface chemistry. Also, the type of targeting, passive or active, and the imaging domain options. The imaging options include optical techniques (fluorescence and bioluminescence) normally using dyes or quantum dots, computed tomography (CT) using heavy metals such as iodine, magnetic resonance imaging (MRI) using superparamagnetic metals like iron oxides and radionuclide imaging (PET and SPECT) using radionuclides [92, 93]. Finally, and probably the most relevant, the active principle, such as drugs, proteins, peptides and genetic material [94]. Table **2** summarizes the diversity of nanomedicine platforms for theranostic purposes.

Moreover, several nanoplatforms for theranostic purposes have intrinsic therapeutic/diagnostics properties, such as gold and/or magnetic nanoparticles or carbon nanotubes due to their capacity to absorb energy and then scatter or emit specific types of therapeutic/diagnostic signals, such as ultrasound heat, Raman or fluorescent signals [103]. Still, one must be very careful when selecting a type of nanovector for theranostic purposes, since these must be able to be functionalized with imaging contrast, therapeutic cargo and targeting elements while retaining their intrinsic properties [104]. The rational design of gene therapy carriers for theranostic applications should consider 1) the genetic material loading capability; 2) transporting the cargo through cellular barriers without triggering immune responses; 3) deliver the cargo into cell nuclei/cytoplasm; 4) allow the transportation of a detection component for noninvasive imaging and visualization of the entire process in real time, without degrading itself or the transported cargo; and 5) provide colloidal stability and functional groups (*e.g.*, *via* polymers, PEG, BSA, *etc.*) to enable bioconjugation to other molecules, such as fluorescent labels and targeting ligands [105, 106].

3.1. Imaging Techniques

Imaging with contrast agents (both molecular- and nanoparticle-based) is a powerful technique to characterize biological processes at (sub)cellular level both *in vivo* as *in vitro*, which is crucial for an effective theranostic system. Exploiting the disease state *via* specific targeting and the help of contrast agents or molecular probes, allows the evaluation of the effectiveness and specificity of a given treatment in real time. Semiconductor nanoparticle-based contrast agents (*e.g.*, quantum dots) have multiple advantages over their chemical-based fluorescent and bioluminescent probes counterparts. The major benefit is that semiconductor NPs do not bleach over time and their decay does not decline over extended use. Other imaging modalities can be used in theranostic systems, nevertheless conjugation of the imaging agent must not interfere with the particle system and its intrinsic properties, and *vice-versa*. Also, one requires a sufficient accumulation of the imaging agent at target site, which can be potentiated by the nanovector, due its size, and disease state-specific targeting.

Table 2. Studies on theranostic nanomedicine platforms for cancer management.

Type of Theranostic System	Material(s)	Application	Experimental Approach	Therapeutic Agent	Imaging Agent	Targeting Agent	Ref.
Drug-polymer conjugates	HPMA	Prostate cancer targeting tumor angiogenesis	*In vivo* (mice)	^{64}Cu	^{64}Cu	RGDyK	[95]
Polymeric nanoparticles	PLGA/TPGS-COOH	Cancer treatment and diagnosis	*In vitro* (MCF-7 breast cancer cells and NIH-3T3 fibroblasts cells)	Docetaxel	Quantum dots	Folic acid	[96]

(Table 2) cont.....

Type of Theranostic System	Material(s)	Application	Experimental Approach	Therapeutic Agent	Imaging Agent	Targeting Agent	Ref.
Solid lipid nanoparticles	Low-density lipoprotein, Cholesterol	Active targeting to tumor α(v)β(3) integrin receptors	*In vivo* (mice)	Paclitaxel / siRNA	Quantum dots	cRGD	[97]
Dendrimers	Poly(propylene imine)	Image-guided drug delivery and photodynamic therapy	*In vitro* (A2780/AD cancer cells) and *in vivo* (mice)	Phthalocyanines	Phthalocyanines	LHRH	[98]
Liposomes	TPGS, Phospholipids, Cholesterol	Multi-functional platform for high performance in co-delivery of therapeutic and imaging agents	*In vitro* (MCF-7 cells)	Docetaxel	Quantum dots	Folic acid	[99]
Micelles	TPGD and F127 surfactant	Thermotherapy and MRI	*In vivo* (mice)	Iron oxide NPs	Iron oxide NPs	Passive targeting	[100]
Gold nanoparticles	Gold nanoparticles	Cancer imaging and therapy	*In vivo* (mice)	Docetaxel	Gold NPs	CPLGLAGG peptide	[101]
Carbon nanomaterials	SWCNTs	Imaging and photothermal cancer therapy	*In vivo* (mice)	Intrinsic property	Intrinsic property	Passive targeting	[102]

Many imaging agents can be replaced by nanoparticles due to the fact that some inorganic NPs exhibit intrinsic imaging abilities, such as gold NPs for CT, iron oxide NPs for MR and quantum dots for optical imaging. Moreover, multimodal imaging platforms can be developed by the combination of these nanoparticles with different imaging agents by co-encapsulation or conjugation. In addition, traditional organic NPs (*e.g.*, liposomes, micelles, and polymeric NPs) can be used to integrate more than two imaging agents on the surface or in the interior. Therefore, it is possible to make different combinations of multimodal imaging probes. Recently, tri-modal imaging probes for PET/optical/ MRI have also been designed by combining radiometal chelates, such as ^{64}Cu-DOTA and ^{111}In-DOTA, to dual MRI/optical probes [107].

Optical Imaging

This type of imaging uses photons emitted from fluorescent or bioluminescent probes to detect specific biomarkers. It is regarded as an attractive option for imaging due to its high sensitivity, lack of ionizing radiation, ability to image in real time, low cost detection and ability to image the spectrum from visible to near-infrared (NIR) [93]. However, poor tissue penetration, susceptibility to noise due to scattering and potential autofluorescence are some of its drawbacks [108].

In this context, probes include fluorophores, semiconductor fluorescent crystals, lanthanide-based probes and quantum dots [109]. Quantum dots are popular nanomaterials within theranostic nanomedicine due to their advantages over organic dyes. They are able to have their fluorescent properties tuned in number ways [110]. Besides, quantum dots emit highly intense signals, have larger absorption coefficients, high level of brightness and they are photostable [111], [112].

Gold NPs have very attractive applications as contrast agents, because they can be visualized with a great variety of imaging techniques. Due to the strong absorption and scattering of light by AuNPs, the most regarded imaging techniques are based on the interaction between AuNPs and light. AuNPs larger than 20nm can be directly imaged with optical microscopy in phase contrast or differential interference contrast (DIC) mode. On the other hand, smaller AuNPs have been recently reported as capable of emit fluorescence upon photo-excitation thus can be visualized with fluoresce microscopy. Additionally, other methods involving photo-excitation like dark field microscopy, photothermal imaging and photoacoustic imaging can also be used. Besides, the interaction of AuNPs with visible light, they can also interact with electron waves and X-rays, providing them the possibility of being used as contrast agents for TEM and X-ray imaging. Finally, AuNPs can also be radioactively labelled by neutron activation, being in this case detected by gamma radiation [113].

An application of AuNPs regarding optical imaging and therapeutic purposes is described by Cordeiro M. *et al.* with gold nanobeacons for tracking gene silencing in Zebrafish. In this study, the gold nanobeacons where design for silence the enhanced green fluorescent protein (EGFP) mRNA in embryos of a fly-EGFP transgenic zebrafish line. The silencing events are measured by fluorescence imaging, where is noticeable a decrease in the emission of EGFP with a concomitant increase in the emission of gold nanobeacons. The results indicate that the gold nanobeacons simultaneously allow the tracking and localization of the silencing events *via* beacon's emission [114].

Computed Tomography

Computed tomography (CT) provides anatomical information due to differences in the X-ray attenuation that is made by the different biological components. Some of the advantages of CT scans are good spatial resolution while providing a three-dimensional image of the area in interest with good detail and uses less radiation than other techniques [115]. Core-shell nanoparticles, liposomes, gold, dendrimers and bismuth are materials that can be used as CT probes in theranostic platforms.

Over the last decades, AuNPs have gained attention as X-ray contrast agents due to the number of favorable properties, such as the relatively high x-ray attenuation coefficient that gold exhibits (when compared with both barium sulfate and iodine), especially at the energy levels used for clinal CT. Other advantage is the longer vascular retention time when compared with iodinated molecules [116]. Popvtzer *et al.* were able to demonstrate, for the first time, cancer detection at a cellular and molecular level using a standard clinical CT instrument by coupling gold nanoparticles with an antibody targeted to the A9 antigen, which is overexpressed in head and neck cancer cells [117].

Magnetic Resonance Imaging

Magnetic resonance imaging (MRI) is the primary diagnostic technique to obtain high-resolution anatomical images, while providing excellent contrast with resolution under the millimeters. It can also be used for the determination of physicochemical states and even obtain detailed neurological information with functional MRI. It is a non-invasive tool, uses non-ionizing radiation and produces tree-dimensional images. However, the need for lanthanide-based contrast agents, the high costs of the maintenance and the equipment and the impossibility of being used in patients with implants are some of its disadvantages [118].

Magnetic nanoparticles have shown great promise for targeted molecular imaging using MRI. In this regard, SPIONs have been greatly studied, once they provide MR contrast enhancement (*i.e.,* changes in signal intensity) by reduction in both T_1 and T_2 signals and have received FDA approval for use in humans in some clinical applications. The study of Gambarota *et al.* highlights the role of ultra-small iron oxide particles (UIOP) in the characterization of the tumor vasculature in mouse brain by contrast-enhanced MRI [119]. Additionally, MNPs could be used to monitoring treatment-induced cell death. In this case, MNPs were functionalized with the protein Annexin V (which has high affinity to membrane phosphatidylserine that is externalized during the early phase of apoptosis) for apoptosis detection. So, the MNP conjugated with Annexin V would allow non-invasive quantification of the apoptotic response *in vivo* and enable efficient adjustments of therapy [120].

Radionuclide Imaging (PET/SPECT)

Positron emission tomography (PET) and Single-photon emission computed tomography (SPECT) can also be used for diagnostic purposes in theranostic applications.

In SPECT technique a camera is needed in order to detect the dosage of γ radiation, which is emitted by the tissue of interest upon the administration of the radionuclides, such as ^{99m}Tc, ^{131}I and ^{67}Ga that usually are injected in the bloodstream and detected *via* γ radiation [121]. Attaching these radionuclides to a nanoparticle or other carrier platform, that is functionalized with both targeting ligand and therapeutic agent, helps to monitor the site of accumulation of the nanoformulation. PET also uses radionuclides and provides images produced by the emitted γ rays. The radionuclides used in PET scans include ^{111}I, ^{64}Cu and ^{18}F which are more expensive than SPEC nucleotides and have a shorter half-life [122]. The advantages of using PET over SPEC include lower concentration of radionuclides required, higher sensitivity and direct assembly of three-dimensional images. Disadvantages include concerns about using ionizing radiation, spatial resolution limitations, the fact that can only detect one radionuclide at a time, and equipment costs [123].

Multifunctional NPs loaded with two different imaging agents are needed in order to overcome the problem of monitoring drug delivery, drug release and therapeutic efficacy of the drug, once no single imaging modality can provide all information. Peng *et al.* developed a system of multifunctional NPs loaded with the near infrared fluorescence (NIRF) dye (IR-780 iodine) and labeled with the radionuclide rhenium-188 (^{188}Re). In this research, IR-780 iodine dye was used both for NIRF imaging and photothermal therapy. The biodistribution of the dye and the photothermal cancer ablation was investigated through NIRF imaging. In addition, the ^{88}Re-labelled nanoparticles were also noninvasively monitoring by micro-SPECT in order to study the real-time biodistribution and tumor accumulation of the drug carriers [124].

3.2. Therapeutic Nucleic Acids

Nucleic acid-based therapies have become promising strategies for various forms of cancer treatment, more precisely in theranostic applications. RNA therapeutics offers the promise of uniquely targeting the precise sequence of nucleic acids involved in a particular disease with greater specificity, improved potency and lower toxicity. Nanobiotechnology offers a great number of carrier systems that could be used for RNAi delivery purposes, including liposomes, micro/nano-spheres, carbon-nanotubes, lipid-based nanoparticles feasible for biological and medical applications [125, 126]. For example, the incorporation or conjugation of RNA interference (RNAi) molecules in nanoparticles has already been approved for use in the clinics [127].

A small sub-set of targetable diseases cannot be tackled by the inhibitory effects of conventional drugs, generally achieved by blocking their target's function. However, in some diseases, primary proteins do not have enzymatic function or have a conformation that is not accessible to conventional drugs or small molecules, hence the name "non-druggable" targets. Nevertheless, these same "non-druggable" molecules have been efficiently targeted by RNAi approach *in vivo* [128, 129] demonstrating an exclusively allele-specific gene silencing [130, 131]. Additionally, it is more efficient to block the mRNA expression of the target gene than each of its encoded proteins.

RNAi is a naturally occurring mechanism used by cells to regulate gene expression, through small double-stranded RNAs (dsRNAs) in a complementarity-dependent manner. This naturally occurring process, which normally involves multiple families of non-coding RNA regulators, such as miRNAs, siRNA and piwi interacting RNAs (piRNAs), is presumed to protect against pathogenic infections and regulate various biological pathways [132]. Among the endogenous RNA regulators, miRNAs are of utmost relevance since they are involved in the regulation of roughly 30% of the human genes [133, 134].

Small Interfering RNA (siRNA)

siRNA molecules belong to the non-coding RNAs (ncRNAs) family, which include long ncRNAs, broadly defined as 200 nucleotides to 100 kbp ncRNAs [135] and small ncRNAs. The majority of small ncRNAs, such as siRNA and miRNA, have been recognized as having an important role in transcriptional regulation, signaling, post-transcriptional gene signaling and cell communication. The precursors of siRNA are dsRNA molecules that are cleaved in the nucleus by DICER into a double-stranded siRNA with 20-25 nucleotide-long. Then, siRNA binds to AGO2-RISC complex: a combination of RNA-induced silencing complex (RISC) and an endonuclease Argonaut 2 (AGO2) [136]. Once the binding to RISC occurs, the siRNA molecule is unwound into a single-stranded form. After, one of the strands binds to the target mRNA sequence with perfect complementarity and AGO2 cleaves the mRNA sequence. This cleavage triggers the mRNA degradation by exonucleases [137].

Challenges faced by siRNA-based therapies include off-target effects, low efficacy delivery, immune system activation and variable efficacies targeting the same region. The off-target effects could occur due to 1) imperfect complementary-binding to non-targeted mRNAs; or 2) entrance of siRNA into the endogenous miRNA systems that tolerate imperfect binding to target mRNAs outside the miRNA seed region, thereby silencing those targets. Despite these drawbacks, there are 26 different siRNAs tested in more than 50 clinical trials against numerous diseases, including age-related muscular degeneration (AMD), diabetic macular edema (DME), hypercholesteremia, glaucoma and human solid tumor (melanoma) [138].

Interestingly, only but a few of these strategies rely on nanoscale carriers. Examples of siRNA applications using NPs as vectors include: 1) the delivery of siRNA specific to cyclin CD-1 by liposomes functionalized with monoclonal antibodies *in vivo* to target leukocytes [139] and 2) Polymeric nanoparticles coated with integrin ligand RGD loaded with siRNA against endothelial cells during angiogenesis [140]. Nevertheless, there are plenty of conceptual proposals that have yet leave the lab and reach the readiness point to be translated to the clinics.

Child, Hernandez and Conde *et al.* demonstrated an example of siRNA as a therapeutic tool. In this work, gold nanoparticle-siRNA conjugates mediate *c-myc* oncogene knockdown at RNA and protein levels in HeLa cells [141]. Also, Conde *et al.* demonstrated the triggering of apoptotic pathways for enhanced cancer-cell killing through RNAi-based glyconanoparticles [142].

MicroRNAs (miRNAs)

miRNAs are conserved single-stranded RNA molecules with 19-25 nucleotides in length and are transcribed by RNA polymerase II [143]. Several studies demonstrate their differential expression in multiple types of cancer cells [144, 145]. Their application as therapeutic agents rely on targeting: oncogenes or other genes involved in their expression. For theranostic purposes, miRNA can be delivered to target cells by targeted nanoparticle systems, such as liposomes for delivery of miR-34a into metastatic melanoma [146] and gold NPs loaded with miR-29b for delivery into HeLa cells [147].

In a similar manner to siRNAs, miRNAs silence gene expression post-transcriptionally [148]. The precursors of miRNA are naturally encoded in the genome, but miRNAs can also be synthetized for therapeutic purposes. At cell level, RNA polymerase II transcribes the primary miRNA (pri-miRNA), then the ribonuclease DROSHA cleaves it, leading to the miRNA precursor (pre-miRNA). Finally, in cytoplasm the RNase III enzyme Dicer cleaves pre-miRNA generating the miRNA. Commonly, miRNAs target mRNAs with imperfect complementarity and suppress their translation, which results in lower expression levels of the corresponding proteins [159]. The 8 nucleotide-long sequence in the 5' region of miRNA is known as seed sequence, which is responsible for miRNA targeting. This sequence has in fact been used in bioinformatics for miRNA target prediction [150]. Due to the imperfect base-paring, a single miRNA molecule can target several mRNAs [151]. Still, the same drawbacks mentioned for siRNA application are also valid for miRNA.

Antisense Oligonucleotides

Antisense oligonucleotides, or ASOs, are DNA/RNA sequences with 15-25 nucleotide-long designed to bind *via* Watson-Crick hybridization, with complementary RNA targets, ultimately facilitating their degradation. ASO technology provided the first-based approach to disrupting gene expression and it has been used in knockdown experiments, target validation and drug therapy. In fact, ASOs are very stable at a wide range of temperature, highly soluble in water and typically are safer than RNAi molecules [152].

ASOs must be able to cross the cell membrane to bind to the RNA target either in the nucleus (*i.e.,* pre-mRNA, mRNA, pre-miRNA) or cytoplasm (*i.e.,* miRNA, mRNA) [153]. ASOs mechanism of action varies with the part of RNA molecule that is targeted and with its own chemical and designing properties. The mRNA sequences targeted by ASOs are chosen based in their biding accessibility.

The two types of ASOs that are mostly used are double-stranded ASOs, which uses RISC complex to degrade the target RNA, and single-stranded ASOs that silence gene expression by a variety of mechanisms including: 1) inhibition of 5' cap formation; 2) steric block of protein formation; 3) inhibition or alteration of RNA splicing; and 4) activation of RNase H that degrades the target RNA [154 - 156].

The work performed by Vinhas R. *et al.* is an example of ASOs technology for cancer therapy. In the present example, the AuNPs functionalized with antisense oligonucleotides, more precisely ssDNA, targeted *BCR-ABL1* chimeric gene *in vitro*. *BCR-ABL1* gene encode for a constitutively active tyrosine kinase that plays the central role in leukemogenesis. The AuNP@ssDNA aims both the silencing of the oncogene and an enhancement in the efficacy of the drug used in the conventional treatment [157].

Table 3. RNAi-based NPs for systemic administration.

Delivery System	Nanoparticle Formulation	Targeting Agent	Target Tissue	Ref.
Lipid-based NPs / Lipoplexes	DOPC liposomes	EPR	Ovarium cancer	[158]
Cationic lipid-based NPs	SNALP	MPS	Liver	[73, 159, 160]
Lipoids	Epoxide-based NPs	MPS	Liver	[161, 162]
Polyplexes	JetPEI/LNA-siRNA polyplex	Aggregation induced retention, Mucoadhesion	Lung, liver and kidney	[163]

(Table 3) cont.....

Delivery System	Nanoparticle Formulation	Targeting Agent	Target Tissue	Ref.
Carbon nanotubes	To17-SWCNTs	MPS	Liver	[164]
Aptamer /NPs	RNA A10/siRNA NPs	PSMA-targeted aptamer	Prostate cancer cells	[165, 166]

Gene Editing via CRISPR

Genome editing (also called gene editing) comprises a group of technologies to change an organism's DNA. These technologies allow genetic material to be added, removed, or altered at particular loci in the genome. One of the most widespread genome editing technologies is CRISPR-Cas9 - clustered regularly interspaced short palindromic repeats and CRISPR-associated protein 9 [167, 168]. The CRISPR-Cas9 strategy was adapted from a naturally occurring system in bacteria, which capture pieces of DNA from infecting viruses and use them to create DNA sections known as CRISPR arrays. The CRISPR arrays allow the bacteria to "remember" those viruses or closely related ones, in a similar way to that of our immune system. If the viruses attack again, the bacteria produce RNA segments from the CRISPR arrays to target the viruses' DNA, followed by Cas9 or a similar enzyme to cut the DNA apart, thus hindering the virus.

Therapeutic use of CRISPR-Cas9 strategy relies on the use of small pieces of RNA with a short "guide" sequence that hybridizes to a specific target sequence in the genome [169, 170]. This RNA also binds to the Cas9 enzyme, which is processed and used to recognize the DNA sequence, allowing the Cas9 enzyme to cut the DNA sequence at the targeted location. Although Cas9 is the enzyme that is used most often, other enzymes (*e.g.* Cpf1) can also be used. Once the genomic DNA is cut, the cell's own DNA repair machinery will add or delete fragments or replace with a customized DNA sequence. Several approaches using nanotechnology-based delivery systems have been proposed for the delivery of the CRISPR-Cas9 machinery to the cells. Currently, the same vectors used for traditional RNAi approaches have been used for CRISPR-Cas9, such as polysaccharide nanoparticles, cationic liposome nanoparticles, calcium phosphate nanoparticles and nanoneedle [171, 172]. One of the biggest challenges to efficient application of CRISPR-Cas9 strategy is the proteolytic instability and poor membrane permeability of genome-editing proteins, which require novel platforms to assemble protein into nanoparticles for intracellular delivery.

Genome editing is considered a great tool to edit abnormal genomic *loci* and provide for a normal DNA fragment to replace the deleterious gene that causes disease. However, one concern with CRISPR-Cas9 technology is that it might make accidental cuts to other parts of the genome that are not being targeted, thus introducing errors to the genome with widespread amplification in tissues [173].

The CRISPR-Cas9 strategy has also raised several ethical concerns since it is capable to directly alter the human genome. Most genome editing efforts are limited to somatic cells, which are not passed from one generation to the next. However, changes made to genes in germline cells or in the genes of an embryo could be passed to future generations.

4. HOW FAR FROM THE CLINICS ARE NANOTHERANOSTICS IN GENE DELIVERY

Despite the potential of nanotheranostics for gene delivery, there are still a multitude of barriers to successful clinical translation. Viral-based vectors have been used for clinical gene therapy due to their efficient transduction, but face several obstacles, such as high adverse side-effects and costs. Developing safe and effective non-viral gene delivery platforms is an utmost need. Among these non-viral gene delivery platforms, NPs-based delivery systems have been in the forefront towards effective gene therapy. Since 2010 when the first clinical trial for gene therapy was achieved several NPs-based gene delivery systems have entered clinical trials (for recent reviews see [21, 174]. However, some of those clinical trials failed to achieve successful endpoints and none of these gene-based nanotherapeutics has been approved by the FDA. Understanding the molecular basis of target diseases, key limiting steps in effective delivering and gene therapy such as extracellular and intracellular barriers, nucleic acids stability and availability, immune system reactivity, delivery routes are in the forefront of challenges towards the clinical progress of nanotheranostics in gene delivery. Efforts to improve targeted delivery strategies of nanomedicines to the desired tissues for optimal therapeutic efficacy with reduced side effects are still needed. But, if successful, these systems will allow synergies between diagnosis and therapy that may be used in combination with drug, hyperthermia, immunotherapy and others. More efforts should be directed also at the effective scale-up of nanomedicines synthesis, assess their long-term toxicity and the creation of regulatory methodologies for nanotheranostics. Only when these challenges are surpassed, may nanotechnology be at the patient's bedside for an effective and personalized therapy.

CONSENT FOR PUBLICATION

Not applicable.

CONFLICT OF INTEREST

The authors confirm that the contents of this chapter have no conflict of interest.

ACKNOWLEDGEMENTS

Declared none.

REFERENCES

[1]   Bray F, Ferlay J, Soerjomataram I, Siegel RL, Torre LA, Jemal A. Global cancer statistics 2018: GLOBOCAN estimates of incidence and mortality worldwide for 36 cancers in 185 countries. CA Cancer J Clin 2018; 68(6): 394-424.
[http://dx.doi.org/10.3322/caac.21492] [PMID: 30207593]

[2]   Brayden DJ. Controlled release technologies for drug delivery. Drug Discov Today 2003; 8(21): 976-8.
[http://dx.doi.org/10.1016/S1359-6446(03)02874-5] [PMID: 14643159]

[3]   Keles E, Song Y, Du D, Dong WJ, Lin Y. Recent progress in nanomaterials for gene delivery applications. Biomater Sci 2016; 4(9): 1291-309.
[http://dx.doi.org/10.1039/C6BM00441E] [PMID: 27480033]

[4]   Torchilin VP. Targeted pharmaceutical nanocarriers for cancer therapy and imaging. AAPS J 2007; 9(2): E128-47.
[http://dx.doi.org/10.1208/aapsj0902015] [PMID: 17614355]

[5]   Somia N, Verma IM. Gene therapy: trials and tribulations. Nat Rev Genet 2000; 1(2): 91-9.
[http://dx.doi.org/10.1038/35038533] [PMID: 11253666]

[6]   Edelstein ML, Abedi MR, Wixon J. Gene therapy clinical trials worldwide to 2007--an update. J Gene Med 2007; 9(10): 833-42.
[http://dx.doi.org/10.1002/jgm.1100] [PMID: 17721874]

[7]   Kaczmarek JC, Kowalski PS, Anderson DG. Advances in the delivery of RNA therapeutics: from concept to clinical reality. Genome Med 2017; 9(1): 60.
[http://dx.doi.org/10.1186/s13073-017-0450-0] [PMID: 28655327]

[8]   Evers MM, Toonen LJ, van Roon-Mom WM. Antisense oligonucleotides in therapy for neurodegenerative disorders. Adv Drug Deliv Rev 2015; 87: 90-103.
[http://dx.doi.org/10.1016/j.addr.2015.03.008] [PMID: 25797014]

[9]   Chery J. RNA therapeutics: RNAi and antisense mechanisms and clinical applications. Postdoc J 2016; 4(7): 35-50.
[http://dx.doi.org/10.14304/SURYA.JPR.V4N7.5] [PMID: 27570789]

[10]   Whitehead KA, Langer R, Anderson DG. Knocking down barriers: advances in siRNA delivery. Nat Rev Drug Discov 2009; 8(2): 129-38.
[http://dx.doi.org/10.1038/nrd2742] [PMID: 19180106]

[11]   Muratovska A, Eccles MR. Conjugate for efficient delivery of short interfering RNA (siRNA) into mammalian cells. FEBS Lett 2004; 558(1-3): 63-8.
[http://dx.doi.org/10.1016/S0014-5793(03)01505-9] [PMID: 14759517]

[12]   Salsman J, Dellaire G. Precision genome editing in the CRISPR era. Biochem Cell Biol 2017; 95(2): 187-201.
[http://dx.doi.org/10.1139/bcb-2016-0137] [PMID: 28177771]

[13]   Christidi E, Huang HM, Brunham LR. CRISPR/Cas9-mediated genome editing in human stem cell-derived cardiomyocytes: Applications for cardiovascular disease modelling and cardiotoxicity screening. Drug Discov Today Technol 2018; 28: 13-21.
[http://dx.doi.org/10.1016/j.ddtec.2018.06.002] [PMID: 30205876]

[14]   Carroll D. Progress and prospects: zinc-finger nucleases as gene therapy agents. Gene Ther 2008; 15(22): 1463-8.

[http://dx.doi.org/10.1038/gt.2008.145] [PMID: 18784746]

[15]   Gaj T, Gersbach CA, Barbas CF III. ZFN, TALEN, and CRISPR/Cas-based methods for genome engineering. Trends Biotechnol 2013; 31(7): 397-405.
[http://dx.doi.org/10.1016/j.tibtech.2013.04.004] [PMID: 23664777]

[16]   Wright DA, Li T, Yang B, Spalding MH. TALEN-mediated genome editing: prospects and perspectives. Biochem J 2014; 462(1): 15-24.
[http://dx.doi.org/10.1042/BJ20140295] [PMID: 25057889]

[17]   Van Tendeloo VF, Van Broeckhoven C, Berneman ZN. Gene therapy: principles and applications to hematopoietic cells. Leukemia 2001; 15(4): 523-44.
[http://dx.doi.org/10.1038/sj.leu.2402085] [PMID: 11368355]

[18]   Adler AF, Leong KW. Emerging links between surface nanotechnology and endocytosis: impact on nonviral gene delivery. Nano Today 2010; 5(6): 553-69.
[http://dx.doi.org/10.1016/j.nantod.2010.10.007] [PMID: 21383869]

[19]   Mintzer MA, Simanek EE. Nonviral vectors for gene delivery. Chem Rev 2009; 109(2): 259-302.
[http://dx.doi.org/10.1021/cr800409e] [PMID: 19053809]

[20]   Alexiou C, Jurgons R, Parak F, Weyh T, Wolf B, Iro H. Applications of Nanotechnology in Medicine. 4th IEEE Conference on Nanotechnology 2004, Munich: Germany 2004, pp. 233-235.
[http://dx.doi.org/10.1109/NANO.2004.1392308]

[21]   Chen H, Zhang W, Zhu G, Xie J, Chen X. Rethinking cancer nanotheranostics. Nat Rev Mater 2017; 2: 17024.
[http://dx.doi.org/10.1038/natrevmats.2017.24] [PMID: 29075517]

[22]   Schlenk F, Grund S, Fischer D. Recent developments and perspectives on gene therapy using synthetic vectors. Ther Deliv 2013; 4(1): 95-113.
[http://dx.doi.org/10.4155/tde.12.128] [PMID: 23323783]

[23]   Alexis F, Pridgen E, Molnar LK, Farokhzad OC. Factors affecting the clearance and biodistribution of polymeric nanoparticles. Mol Pharm 2008; 5(4): 505-15.
[http://dx.doi.org/10.1021/mp800051m] [PMID: 18672949]

[24]   Jiang S, Eltoukhy AA, Love KT, Langer R, Anderson DG. Lipidoid-coated iron oxide nanoparticles for efficient DNA and siRNA delivery. Nano Lett 2013; 13(3): 1059-64.
[http://dx.doi.org/10.1021/nl304287a] [PMID: 23394319]

[25]   Marchini C, Pozzi D, Montani M, *et al.* Tailoring lipoplex composition to the lipid composition of plasma membrane: a Trojan horse for cell entry? Langmuir 2010; 26(17): 13867-73.
[http://dx.doi.org/10.1021/la1023899] [PMID: 20669909]

[26]   Cardarelli F, Pozzi D, Bifone A, Marchini C, Caracciolo G. Cholesterol-dependent macropinocytosis and endosomal escape control the transfection efficiency of lipoplexes in CHO living cells. Mol Pharm 2012; 9(2): 334-40.
[http://dx.doi.org/10.1021/mp200374e] [PMID: 22196199]

[27]   Kesharwani P, Iyer AK. Recent advances in dendrimer-based nanovectors for tumor-targeted drug and gene delivery. Drug Discov Today 2015; 20(5): 536-47.
[http://dx.doi.org/10.1016/j.drudis.2014.12.012] [PMID: 25555748]

[28]   Kommareddy S, Amiji M. Poly(ethylene glycol)-modified thiolated gelatin nanoparticles for glutathione-responsive intracellular DNA delivery. Nanomedicine (Lond) 2007; 3(1): 32-42.
[http://dx.doi.org/10.1016/j.nano.2006.11.005] [PMID: 17379167]

[29]   Betancourt T, Byrne JD, Sunaryo N, *et al.* PEGylation strategies for active targeting of PLA/PLGA nanoparticles. J Biomed Mater Res A 2009; 91(1): 263-76.
[http://dx.doi.org/10.1002/jbm.a.32247] [PMID: 18980197]

[30]   Grigsby CL, Leong KW. Balancing protection and release of DNA: tools to address a bottleneck of

non-viral gene delivery. J R Soc Interface 2010; 7 (Suppl. 1): S67-82.
[http://dx.doi.org/10.1098/rsif.2009.0260] [PMID: 19734186]

[31]   Belting M, Sandgren S, Wittrup A. Nuclear delivery of macromolecules: barriers and carriers. Adv Drug Deliv Rev 2005; 57(4): 505-27.
[http://dx.doi.org/10.1016/j.addr.2004.10.004] [PMID: 15722161]

[32]   Soenen SJ, De Cuyper M. Assessing iron oxide nanoparticle toxicity *in vitro*: current status and future prospects. Nanomedicine (Lond) 2010; 5(8): 1261-75.
[http://dx.doi.org/10.2217/nnm.10.106] [PMID: 21039201]

[33]   Corvo ML, Mendo AS, Figueiredo S, *et al.* Liposomes as delivery system of a Sn(IV) complex for cancer therapy. Pharm Res 2016; 33(6): 1351-8.
[http://dx.doi.org/10.1007/s11095-016-1876-6] [PMID: 27033349]

[34]   Ma B, Zhang S, Jiang H, Zhao B, Lv H. Lipoplex morphologies and their influences on transfection efficiency in gene delivery. J Control Release 2007; 123(3): 184-94.
[http://dx.doi.org/10.1016/j.jconrel.2007.08.022] [PMID: 17913276]

[35]   Gujrati M, Malamas A, Shin T, Jin E, Sun Y, Lu ZR. Multifunctional cationic lipid-based nanoparticles facilitate endosomal escape and reduction-triggered cytosolic siRNA release. Mol Pharm 2014; 11(8): 2734-44.
[http://dx.doi.org/10.1021/mp400787s] [PMID: 25020033]

[36]   Pedersen N, Hansen S, Heydenreich AV, Kristensen HG, Poulsen HS. Solid lipid nanoparticles can effectively bind DNA, streptavidin and biotinylated ligands. Eur J Pharm Biopharm 2006; 62(2): 155-62.
[http://dx.doi.org/10.1016/j.ejpb.2005.09.003] [PMID: 16290122]

[37]   Thiruganesh R, Devi S. Solid lipid nanoparticle and nanoparticle lipid carrier for controlled drug delivery – a review of state of art and recent advances. Int J Nanopart 2010; 3: 32.
[http://dx.doi.org/10.1504/IJNP.2010.033220]

[38]   Tabatt K, Kneuer C, Sameti M, *et al.* Transfection with different colloidal systems: comparison of solid lipid nanoparticles and liposomes. J Control Release 2004; 97(2): 321-32.
[http://dx.doi.org/10.1016/j.jconrel.2004.02.029] [PMID: 15196759]

[39]   Choi SH, Jin SE, Lee MK, *et al.* Novel cationic solid lipid nanoparticles enhanced p53 gene transfer to lung cancer cells. Eur J Pharm Biopharm 2008; 68(3): 545-54.
[http://dx.doi.org/10.1016/j.ejpb.2007.07.011] [PMID: 17881199]

[40]   Ishida T, Ichikawa T, Ichihara M, Sadzuka Y, Kiwada H. Effect of the physicochemical properties of initially injected liposomes on the clearance of subsequently injected PEGylated liposomes in mice. J Control Release 2004; 95(3): 403-12.
[http://dx.doi.org/10.1016/j.jconrel.2003.12.011] [PMID: 15023452]

[41]   Yu W, Liu C, Ye J, Zou W, Zhang N, Xu W. Novel cationic SLN containing a synthesized single-tailed lipid as a modifier for gene delivery. Nanotechnology 2009; 20(21): 215102.
[http://dx.doi.org/10.1088/0957-4484/20/21/215102] [PMID: 19423923]

[42]   Kwon SM, Nam HY, Nam T, *et al. In vivo* time-dependent gene expression of cationic lipid-based emulsion as a stable and biocompatible non-viral gene carrier. J Control Release 2008; 128(1): 89-97.
[http://dx.doi.org/10.1016/j.jconrel.2008.02.004] [PMID: 18384902]

[43]   Nam HY, Park JH, Kim K, Kwon IC, Jeong SY. Lipid-based emulsion system as non-viral gene carriers. Arch Pharm Res 2009; 32(5): 639-46.
[http://dx.doi.org/10.1007/s12272-009-1500-y] [PMID: 19471876]

[44]   Choi WJ, Kim JK, Choi SH, Park JS, Ahn WS, Kim CK. Low toxicity of cationic lipid-based emulsion for gene transfer. Biomaterials 2004; 25(27): 5893-903.
[http://dx.doi.org/10.1016/j.biomaterials.2004.01.031] [PMID: 15172502]

[45]   Torchilin VP. Cell penetrating peptide-modified pharmaceutical nanocarriers for intracellular drug and

gene delivery. Biopolymers 2008; 90(5): 604-10.
[http://dx.doi.org/10.1002/bip.20989] [PMID: 18381624]

[46]   Peer D, Karp JM, Hong S, Farokhzad OC, Margalit R, Langer R. Nanocarriers as an emerging platform for cancer therapy. Nat Nanotechnol 2007; 2(12): 751-60.
[http://dx.doi.org/10.1038/nnano.2007.387] [PMID: 18654426]

[47]   Liu CH, Yu SY. Cationic nanoemulsions as non-viral vectors for plasmid DNA delivery. Colloids Surf B Biointerfaces 2010; 79(2): 509-15.
[http://dx.doi.org/10.1016/j.colsurfb.2010.05.026] [PMID: 20541375]

[48]   Zhang S, Xu Y, Wang B, Qiao W, Liu D, Li Z. Cationic compounds used in lipoplexes and polyplexes for gene delivery. J Control Release 2004; 100(2): 165-80.
[http://dx.doi.org/10.1016/j.jconrel.2004.08.019] [PMID: 15544865]

[49]   Williams DS, Pijpers IAB, Ridolfo R, van Hest JCM. Controlling the morphology of copolymeric vectors for next generation nanomedicine. J Control Release 2017; 259: 29-39.
[http://dx.doi.org/10.1016/j.jconrel.2017.02.030] [PMID: 28257992]

[50]   El-Sayed IH, Huang X, El-Sayed MA. Selective laser photo-thermal therapy of epithelial carcinoma using anti-EGFR antibody conjugated gold nanoparticles. Cancer Lett 2006; 239(1): 129-35.
[http://dx.doi.org/10.1016/j.canlet.2005.07.035] [PMID: 16198049]

[51]   Midoux P, Pichon C, Yaouanc JJ, Jaffrès PA. Chemical vectors for gene delivery: a current review on polymers, peptides and lipids containing histidine or imidazole as nucleic acids carriers. Br J Pharmacol 2009; 157(2): 166-78.
[http://dx.doi.org/10.1111/j.1476-5381.2009.00288.x] [PMID: 19459843]

[52]   Al-Dosari MS, Gao X. Nonviral gene delivery: principle, limitations, and recent progress. AAPS J 2009; 11(4): 671-81.
[http://dx.doi.org/10.1208/s12248-009-9143-y] [PMID: 19834816]

[53]   Hara T, Tan Y, Huang L. *In vivo* gene delivery to the liver using reconstituted chylomicron remnants as a novel nonviral vector. Proc Natl Acad Sci USA 1997; 94(26): 14547-52.
[http://dx.doi.org/10.1073/pnas.94.26.14547] [PMID: 9405650]

[54]   Pedrosa P, Heuer-Jungemann A, Kanaras AG, Fernandes AR, Baptista PV. Potentiating angiogenesis arrest *in vivo via* laser irradiation of peptide functionalised gold nanoparticles. J Nanobiotechnology 2017; 15(1): 85.
[http://dx.doi.org/10.1186/s12951-017-0321-2] [PMID: 29162137]

[55]   Strand SP, Lelu S, Reitan NK, de Lange Davies C, Artursson P, Vårum KM. Molecular design of chitosan gene delivery systems with an optimized balance between polyplex stability and polyplex unpacking. Biomaterials 2010; 31(5): 975-87.
[http://dx.doi.org/10.1016/j.biomaterials.2009.09.102] [PMID: 19857892]

[56]   Saranya N, Moorthi A, Saravanan S, Devi MP, Selvamurugan N. Chitosan and its derivatives for gene delivery. Int J Biol Macromol 2011; 48(2): 234-8.
[http://dx.doi.org/10.1016/j.ijbiomac.2010.11.013] [PMID: 21134396]

[57]   Wasungu L, Hoekstra D. Cationic lipids, lipoplexes and intracellular delivery of genes. J Control Release 2006; 116(2): 255-64.
[http://dx.doi.org/10.1016/j.jconrel.2006.06.024] [PMID: 16914222]

[58]   Liu C, Zhang N. Nanoparticles in gene therapy principles, prospects, and challenges. Prog Mol Biol Transl Sci 2011; 104: 509-62.
[http://dx.doi.org/10.1016/B978-0-12-416020-0.00013-9] [PMID: 22093228]

[59]   Zhi D, Zhang S, Wang B, Zhao Y, Yang B, Yu S. Transfection efficiency of cationic lipids with different hydrophobic domains in gene delivery. Bioconjug Chem 2010; 21(4): 563-77.
[http://dx.doi.org/10.1021/bc900393r] [PMID: 20121120]

[60]   Montier T, Benvegnu T, Jaffrès PA, Yaouanc JJ, Lehn P. Progress in cationic lipid-mediated gene

transfection: a series of bio-inspired lipids as an example. Curr Gene Ther 2008; 8(5): 296-312.
[http://dx.doi.org/10.2174/156652308786070989] [PMID: 18855628]

[61] Mével M, Kamaly N, Carmona S, *et al.* DODAG; a versatile new cationic lipid that mediates efficient delivery of pDNA and siRNA. J Control Release 2010; 143(2): 222-32.
[http://dx.doi.org/10.1016/j.jconrel.2009.12.001] [PMID: 19969034]

[62] Li W, Szoka FC Jr. Lipid-based nanoparticles for nucleic acid delivery. Pharm Res 2007; 24(3): 438-49.
[http://dx.doi.org/10.1007/s11095-006-9180-5] [PMID: 17252188]

[63] Ajmani PS, Hughes JA. 3β [N-(N',N'-dimethylaminoethane)-carbamoyl] cholesterol (DC-Chol-mediated gene delivery to primary rat neurons: characterization and mechanism. Neurochem Res 1999; 24(5): 699-703.
[http://dx.doi.org/10.1023/A:1021012727796] [PMID: 10344600]

[64] Martin B, Sainlos M, Aissaoui A, *et al.* The design of cationic lipids for gene delivery. Curr Pharm Des 2005; 11(3): 375-94.
[http://dx.doi.org/10.2174/1381612053382133] [PMID: 15723632]

[65] Elouahabi A, Ruysschaert JM. Formation and intracellular trafficking of lipoplexes and polyplexes. Mol Ther 2005; 11(3): 336-47.
[http://dx.doi.org/10.1016/j.ymthe.2004.12.006] [PMID: 15727930]

[66] Makadia HK, Siegel SJ. Poly lactic-co-glycolic acid (PLGA) as biodegradable controlled drug delivery carrier. Polymers (Basel) 2011; 3(3): 1377-97.
[http://dx.doi.org/10.3390/polym3031377] [PMID: 22577513]

[67] Wong S, Pelet J, Putnam D. Polymer systems for gene delivery—Past, present, and future. Prog Polym Sci 2007; 32: 799-837.
[http://dx.doi.org/10.1016/j.progpolymsci.2007.05.007]

[68] Wang D, Robinson DR, Kwon GS, Samuel J. Encapsulation of plasmid DNA in biodegradable poly(D, L-lactic-co-glycolic acid) microspheres as a novel approach for immunogene delivery. J Control Release 1999; 57(1): 9-18.
[http://dx.doi.org/10.1016/S0168-3659(98)00099-6] [PMID: 9863034]

[69] Schaffer DV, Fidelman NA, Dan N, Lauffenburger DA. Vector unpacking as a potential barrier for receptor-mediated polyplex gene delivery. Biotechnol Bioeng 2000; 67(5): 598-606.
[http://dx.doi.org/10.1002/(SICI)1097-0290(20000305)67:5<598::AID-BIT10>3.0.CO;2-G] [PMID: 10649234]

[70] Mehier-Humbert S, Guy RH. Physical methods for gene transfer: improving the kinetics of gene delivery into cells. Adv Drug Deliv Rev 2005; 57(5): 733-53.
[http://dx.doi.org/10.1016/j.addr.2004.12.007] [PMID: 15757758]

[71] Plank C, Schillinger U, Scherer F, *et al.* The magnetofection method: using magnetic force to enhance gene delivery. Biol Chem 2003; 384(5): 737-47.
[http://dx.doi.org/10.1515/BC.2003.082] [PMID: 12817470]

[72] Ulasov AV, Khramtsov YV, Trusov GA, Rosenkranz AA, Sverdlov ED, Sobolev AS. Properties of PEI-based polyplex nanoparticles that correlate with their transfection efficacy. Mol Ther 2011; 19(1): 103-12.
[http://dx.doi.org/10.1038/mt.2010.233] [PMID: 21045811]

[73] Song H, Wang G, He B, *et al.* Cationic lipid-coated PEI/DNA polyplexes with improved efficiency and reduced cytotoxicity for gene delivery into mesenchymal stem cells. Int J Nanomed 2012; 7: 4637-48.
[PMID: 22942645]

[74] Xu Q, Leong J, Chua QY, *et al.* Combined modality doxorubicin-based chemotherapy and chitosan-mediated p53 gene therapy using double-walled microspheres for treatment of human hepatocellular

carcinoma. Biomaterials 2013; 34(21): 5149-62.
[http://dx.doi.org/10.1016/j.biomaterials.2013.03.044] [PMID: 23578555]

[75] Kabanov AV, Kabanov VA. DNA complexes with polycations for the delivery of genetic material into cells. Bioconjug Chem 1995; 6(1): 7-20.
[http://dx.doi.org/10.1021/bc00031a002] [PMID: 7711106]

[76] Tros de Ilarduya C, Sun Y, Düzgüneş N. Gene delivery by lipoplexes and polyplexes. Eur J Pharm Sci 2010; 40(3): 159-70.
[http://dx.doi.org/10.1016/j.ejps.2010.03.019] [PMID: 20359532]

[77] Insua I, Wilkinson A, Fernandez-Trillo F. Polyion complex (PIC) particles: Preparation and biomedical applications. Eur Polym J 2016; 81: 198-215.
[http://dx.doi.org/10.1016/j.eurpolymj.2016.06.003] [PMID: 27524831]

[78] Henke E, Perk J, Vider J, *et al.* Peptide-conjugated antisense oligonucleotides for targeted inhibition of a transcriptional regulator *in vivo*. Nat Biotechnol 2008; 26(1): 91-100.
[http://dx.doi.org/10.1038/nbt1366] [PMID: 18176556]

[79] Wang Y, Li Z, Weber TJ, *et al. In situ* live cell sensing of multiple nucleotides exploiting DNA/RNA aptamers and graphene oxide nanosheets. Anal Chem 2013; 85(14): 6775-82.
[http://dx.doi.org/10.1021/ac400858g] [PMID: 23758346]

[80] Ho YP, Leong KW. Quantum dot-based theranostics. Nanoscale 2010; 2(1): 60-8.
[http://dx.doi.org/10.1039/B9NR00178F] [PMID: 20648364]

[81] Yong KT, Roy I, Ding H, Bergey EJ, Prasad PN. Biocompatible near-infrared quantum dots as ultrasensitive probes for long-term *in vivo* imaging applications. Small 2009; 5(17): 1997-2004.
[http://dx.doi.org/10.1002/smll.200900547] [PMID: 19466710]

[82] Qi L, Gao X. Emerging application of quantum dots for drug delivery and therapy. Expert Opin Drug Deliv 2008; 5(3): 263-7.
[http://dx.doi.org/10.1517/17425247.5.3.263] [PMID: 18318649]

[83] Zrazhevskiy P, Sena M, Gao X. Designing multifunctional quantum dots for bioimaging, detection, and drug delivery. Chem Soc Rev 2010; 39(11): 4326-54.
[http://dx.doi.org/10.1039/b915139g] [PMID: 20697629]

[84] Michalet X, Pinaud FF, Bentolila LA, *et al.* Quantum dots for live cells, *in vivo* imaging, and diagnostics. Science 2005; 307(5709): 538-44.
[http://dx.doi.org/10.1126/science.1104274] [PMID: 15681376]

[85] Veiseh O, Gunn JW, Zhang M. Design and fabrication of magnetic nanoparticles for targeted drug delivery and imaging. Adv Drug Deliv Rev 2010; 62(3): 284-304.
[http://dx.doi.org/10.1016/j.addr.2009.11.002] [PMID: 19909778]

[86] Zhang Y, Kohler N, Zhang M. Surface modification of superparamagnetic magnetite nanoparticles and their intracellular uptake. Biomaterials 2002; 23(7): 1553-61.
[http://dx.doi.org/10.1016/S0142-9612(01)00267-8] [PMID: 11922461]

[87] Ghosh P, Han G, De M, Kim CK, Rotello VM. Gold nanoparticles in delivery applications. Adv Drug Deliv Rev 2008; 60(11): 1307-15.
[http://dx.doi.org/10.1016/j.addr.2008.03.016] [PMID: 18555555]

[88] Arvizo R, Bhattacharya R, Mukherjee P. Gold nanoparticles: opportunities and challenges in nanomedicine. Expert Opin Drug Deliv 2010; 7(6): 753-63.
[http://dx.doi.org/10.1517/17425241003777010] [PMID: 20408736]

[89] Gan CW, Chien S, Feng SS. Nanomedicine: enhancement of chemotherapeutical efficacy of docetaxel by using a biodegradable nanoparticle formulation. Curr Pharm Des 2010; 16(21): 2308-20.
[http://dx.doi.org/10.2174/138161210791920487] [PMID: 20618152]

[90] Deveza L, Choi J, Yang F. Therapeutic angiogenesis for treating cardiovascular diseases. Theranostics

2012; 2(8): 801-14.
[http://dx.doi.org/10.7150/thno.4419] [PMID: 22916079]

[91]   Tan YF, Chandrasekharan P, Maity D, *et al.* Multimodal tumor imaging by iron oxides and quantum dots formulated in poly (lactic acid)-D-alpha-tocopheryl polyethylene glycol 1000 succinate nanoparticles. Biomaterials 2011; 32(11): 2969-78.
[http://dx.doi.org/10.1016/j.biomaterials.2010.12.055] [PMID: 21257200]

[92]   Janib SM, Moses AS, MacKay JA. Imaging and drug delivery using theranostic nanoparticles. Adv Drug Deliv Rev 2010; 62(11): 1052-63.
[http://dx.doi.org/10.1016/j.addr.2010.08.004] [PMID: 20709124]

[93]   Xie J, Lee S, Chen X. Nanoparticle-based theranostic agents. Adv Drug Deliv Rev 2010; 62(11): 1064-79.
[http://dx.doi.org/10.1016/j.addr.2010.07.009] [PMID: 20691229]

[94]   Kelkar SS, Reineke TM. Theranostics: combining imaging and therapy. Bioconjug Chem 2011; 22(10): 1879-903.
[http://dx.doi.org/10.1021/bc200151q] [PMID: 21830812]

[95]   Yuan J, Zhang H, Kaur H, Oupicky D, Peng F. Synthesis and characterization of theranostic poly(HPMA)-c(RGDyK)-DOTA-64Cu copolymer targeting tumor angiogenesis: tumor localization visualized by positron emission tomography. Mol Imaging 2013; 12(3): 203-12.
[http://dx.doi.org/10.2310/7290.2012.00038] [PMID: 23490439]

[96]   Pan J, Liu Y, Feng SS. Multifunctional nanoparticles of biodegradable copolymer blend for cancer diagnosis and treatment. Nanomedicine (Lond) 2010; 5(3): 347-60.
[http://dx.doi.org/10.2217/nnm.10.13] [PMID: 20394529]

[97]   Shuhendler AJ, Prasad P, Leung M, Rauth AM, Dacosta RS, Wu XY. A novel solid lipid nanoparticle formulation for active targeting to tumor α(v) β(3) integrin receptors reveals cyclic RGD as a double-edged sword. Adv Healthc Mater 2012; 1(5): 600-8.
[http://dx.doi.org/10.1002/adhm.201200006] [PMID: 23184795]

[98]   Taratula O, Schumann C, Naleway MA, Pang AJ, Chon KJ, Taratula O. A multifunctional theranostic platform based on phthalocyanine-loaded dendrimer for image-guided drug delivery and photodynamic therapy. Mol Pharm 2013; 10(10): 3946-58.
[http://dx.doi.org/10.1021/mp400397t] [PMID: 24020847]

[99]   Muthu MS, Kulkarni SA, Raju A, Feng SS. Theranostic liposomes of TPGS coating for targeted co-delivery of docetaxel and quantum dots. Biomaterials 2012; 33(12): 3494-501.
[http://dx.doi.org/10.1016/j.biomaterials.2012.01.036] [PMID: 22306020]

[100] Chandrasekharan P, Maity D, Yong CX, Chuang KH, Ding J, Feng SS. Vitamin E (D-alph--tocopheryl-co-poly(ethylene glycol) 1000 succinate) micelles-superparamagnetic iron oxide nanoparticles for enhanced thermotherapy and MRI. Biomaterials 2011; 32(24): 5663-72.
[http://dx.doi.org/10.1016/j.biomaterials.2011.04.037] [PMID: 21550654]

[101] Chen WH, Xu XD, Jia HZ, *et al.* Therapeutic nanomedicine based on dual-intelligent functionalized gold nanoparticles for cancer imaging and therapy *in vivo.* Biomaterials 2013; 34(34): 8798-807.
[http://dx.doi.org/10.1016/j.biomaterials.2013.07.084] [PMID: 23932289]

[102] Robinson JT, Welsher K, Tabakman SM, *et al.* High performance *in vivo* near-IR (>1 μm) imaging and photothermal cancer therapy with carbon nanotubes. Nano Res 2010; 3(11): 779-93.
[http://dx.doi.org/10.1007/s12274-010-0045-1] [PMID: 21804931]

[103] Muthu MS, Leong DT, Mei L, Feng SS, Nanotheranostics -. Nanotheranostics - application and further development of nanomedicine strategies for advanced theranostics. Theranostics 2014; 4(6): 660-77.
[http://dx.doi.org/10.7150/thno.8698] [PMID: 24723986]

[104] Cole JT, Holland NB. Multifunctional nanoparticles for use in theranostic applications. Drug Deliv Transl Res 2015; 5(3): 295-309.

[http://dx.doi.org/10.1007/s13346-015-0218-2] [PMID: 25787729]

[105] Liu G, Swierczewska M, Lee S, Chen X. Functional nanoparticles for molecular imaging guided gene delivery. Nano Today 2010; 5(6): 524-39.
[http://dx.doi.org/10.1016/j.nantod.2010.10.005] [PMID: 22473061]

[106] Niu G, Chen X. Noninvasive visualization of microRNA by bioluminescence imaging. Mol Imaging Biol 2009; 11(2): 61-3.
[http://dx.doi.org/10.1007/s11307-008-0190-z] [PMID: 19037611]

[107] Xie J, Chen K, Huang J, *et al.* PET/NIRF/MRI triple functional iron oxide nanoparticles. Biomaterials 2010; 31(11): 3016-22.
[http://dx.doi.org/10.1016/j.biomaterials.2010.01.010] [PMID: 20092887]

[108] Debbage P, Jaschke W. Molecular imaging with nanoparticles: giant roles for dwarf actors. Histochem Cell Biol 2008; 130(5): 845-75.
[http://dx.doi.org/10.1007/s00418-008-0511-y] [PMID: 18825403]

[109] Choi KY, Jeon EJ, Yoon HY, *et al.* Theranostic nanoparticles based on PEGylated hyaluronic acid for the diagnosis, therapy and monitoring of colon cancer. Biomaterials 2012; 33(26): 6186-93.
[http://dx.doi.org/10.1016/j.biomaterials.2012.05.029] [PMID: 22687759]

[110] Medintz IL, Uyeda HT, Goldman ER, Mattoussi H. Quantum dot bioconjugates for imaging, labelling and sensing. Nat Mater 2005; 4(6): 435-46.
[http://dx.doi.org/10.1038/nmat1390] [PMID: 15928695]

[111] Santra S. The potential clinical impact of quantum dots. Nanomedicine (Lond) 2012; 7(5): 623-6.
[http://dx.doi.org/10.2217/nnm.12.45] [PMID: 22630145]

[112] Yong KT, Wang Y, Roy I, *et al.* Preparation of quantum dot/drug nanoparticle formulations for traceable targeted delivery and therapy. Theranostics 2012; 2(7): 681-94.
[http://dx.doi.org/10.7150/thno.3692] [PMID: 22896770]

[113] Sperling RA, Rivera Gil P, Zhang F, Zanella M, Parak WJ. Biological applications of gold nanoparticles. Chem Soc Rev 2008; 37(9): 1896-908.
[http://dx.doi.org/10.1039/b712170a] [PMID: 18762838]

[114] Cordeiro M, Carvalho L, Silva J, Saúde L, Fernandes AR, Baptista PV. Gold nanobeacons for tracking gene silencing in zebrafish. Nanomaterials (Basel) 2017; 7(1): 10.
[http://dx.doi.org/10.3390/nano7010010] [PMID: 28336844]

[115] Shilo M, Reuveni T, Motiei M, Popovtzer R. Nanoparticles as computed tomography contrast agents: current status and future perspectives. Nanomedicine (Lond) 2012; 7(2): 257-69.
[http://dx.doi.org/10.2217/nnm.11.190] [PMID: 22339135]

[116] Cole LE, Ross RD, Tilley JM, Vargo-Gogola T, Roeder RK. Gold nanoparticles as contrast agents in x-ray imaging and computed tomography. Nanomedicine (Lond) 2015; 10(2): 321-41.
[http://dx.doi.org/10.2217/nnm.14.171] [PMID: 25600973]

[117] Reuveni T, Motiei M, Romman Z, Popovtzer A, Popovtzer R. Targeted gold nanoparticles enable molecular CT imaging of cancer: an *in vivo* study. Int J Nanomed 2011; 6: 2859-64.
[PMID: 22131831]

[118] Wang C, Ravi S, Garapati US, *et al.* Multifunctional chitosan magnetic-graphene (CMG) nanoparticles: a theranostic platform for tumor-targeted co-delivery of drugs, genes and MRI contrast agents. J Mater Chem B Mater Biol Med 2013; 1(35): 4396-405.
[http://dx.doi.org/10.1039/c3tb20452a] [PMID: 24883188]

[119] Gambarota G, Leenders W, Maass C, *et al.* Characterisation of tumour vasculature in mouse brain by USPIO contrast-enhanced MRI. Br J Cancer 2008; 98(11): 1784-9.
[http://dx.doi.org/10.1038/sj.bjc.6604389] [PMID: 18506183]

[120] Asín L, Ibarra MR, Tres A, Goya GF. Controlled cell death by magnetic hyperthermia: effects of

exposure time, field amplitude, and nanoparticle concentration. Pharm Res 2012; 29(5): 1319-27.
[http://dx.doi.org/10.1007/s11095-012-0710-z] [PMID: 22362408]

[121] Zanzonico P. Principles of nuclear medicine imaging: planar, SPECT, PET, multi-modality, and autoradiography systems. Radiat Res 2012; 177(4): 349-64.
[http://dx.doi.org/10.1667/RR2577.1] [PMID: 22364319]

[122] Liu Y, Welch MJ. Nanoparticles labeled with positron emitting nuclides: advantages, methods, and applications. Bioconjug Chem 2012; 23(4): 671-82.
[http://dx.doi.org/10.1021/bc200264c] [PMID: 22242601]

[123] Juweid ME, Cheson BD. Positron-emission tomography and assessment of cancer therapy. N Engl J Med 2006; 354(5): 496-507.
[http://dx.doi.org/10.1056/NEJMra050276] [PMID: 16452561]

[124] Peng CL, Shih YH, Lee PC, Hsieh TM, Luo TY, Shieh MJ. Multimodal image-guided photothermal therapy mediated by 188Re-labeled micelles containing a cyanine-type photosensitizer. ACS Nano 2011; 5(7): 5594-607.
[http://dx.doi.org/10.1021/nn201100m] [PMID: 21671580]

[125] Ferrari M. Cancer nanotechnology: opportunities and challenges. Nat Rev Cancer 2005; 5(3): 161-71.
[http://dx.doi.org/10.1038/nrc1566] [PMID: 15738981]

[126] Whitesides GM. The 'right' size in nanobiotechnology. Nat Biotechnol 2003; 21(10): 1161-5.
[http://dx.doi.org/10.1038/nbt872] [PMID: 14520400]

[127] Tiemann K, Rossi JJ. RNAi-based therapeutics-current status, challenges and prospects. EMBO Mol Med 2009; 1(3): 142-51.
[http://dx.doi.org/10.1002/emmm.200900023] [PMID: 20049714]

[128] Zimmermann TS, Lee AC, Akinc A, *et al.* RNAi-mediated gene silencing in non-human primates. Nature 2006; 441(7089): 111-4.
[http://dx.doi.org/10.1038/nature04688] [PMID: 16565705]

[129] Gaudillière B, Shi Y, Bonni A. RNA interference reveals a requirement for myocyte enhancer factor 2A in activity-dependent neuronal survival. J Biol Chem 2002; 277(48): 46442-6.
[http://dx.doi.org/10.1074/jbc.M206653200] [PMID: 12235147]

[130] Miller VM, Xia H, Marrs GL, *et al.* Allele-specific silencing of dominant disease genes. Proc Natl Acad Sci USA 2003; 100(12): 7195-200.
[http://dx.doi.org/10.1073/pnas.1231012100] [PMID: 12782788]

[131] Gonzalez-Alegre P, Bode N, Davidson BL, Paulson HL. Silencing primary dystonia: lentiviral-mediated RNA interference therapy for DYT1 dystonia. J Neurosci 2005; 25(45): 10502-9.
[http://dx.doi.org/10.1523/JNEUROSCI.3016-05.2005] [PMID: 16280588]

[132] Sledz CA, Williams BR. RNA interference in biology and disease. Blood 2005; 106(3): 787-94.
[http://dx.doi.org/10.1182/blood-2004-12-4643] [PMID: 15827131]

[133] Jinek M, Doudna JA. A three-dimensional view of the molecular machinery of RNA interference. Nature 2009; 457(7228): 405-12.
[http://dx.doi.org/10.1038/nature07755] [PMID: 19158786]

[134] Lewis BP, Burge CB, Bartel DP. Conserved seed pairing, often flanked by adenosines, indicates that thousands of human genes are microRNA targets. Cell 2005; 120(1): 15-20.
[http://dx.doi.org/10.1016/j.cell.2004.12.035] [PMID: 15652477]

[135] Jorgensen R. Altered gene expression in plants due to trans interactions between homologous genes. Trends Biotechnol 1990; 8(12): 340-4.
[http://dx.doi.org/10.1016/0167-7799(90)90220-R] [PMID: 1366894]

[136] Meister G. Argonaute proteins: functional insights and emerging roles. Nat Rev Genet 2013; 14(7): 447-59.

[http://dx.doi.org/10.1038/nrg3462] [PMID: 23732335]

[137] Hammond SM, Bernstein E, Beach D, Hannon GJ. An RNA-directed nuclease mediates post-transcriptional gene silencing in Drosophila cells. Nature 2000; 404(6775): 293-6.
[http://dx.doi.org/10.1038/35005107] [PMID: 10749213]

[138] Ozcan G, Ozpolat B, Coleman RL, Sood AK, Lopez-Berestein G. Preclinical and clinical development of siRNA-based therapeutics. Adv Drug Deliv Rev 2015; 87: 108-19.
[http://dx.doi.org/10.1016/j.addr.2015.01.007] [PMID: 25666164]

[139] Peer D, Park EJ, Morishita Y, Carman CV, Shimaoka M. Systemic leukocyte-directed siRNA delivery revealing cyclin D1 as an anti-inflammatory target. Science 2008; 319(5863): 627-30.
[http://dx.doi.org/10.1126/science.1149859] [PMID: 18239128]

[140] Schiffelers RM, Storm G. ICS-283: a system for targeted intravenous delivery of siRNA. Expert Opin Drug Deliv 2006; 3(3): 445-54.
[http://dx.doi.org/10.1517/17425247.3.3.445] [PMID: 16640503]

[141] Child HW, Hernandez Y, Conde J, *et al.* Gold nanoparticle-siRNA mediated oncogene knockdown at RNA and protein level, with associated gene effects. Nanomedicine (Lond) 2015; 10(16): 2513-25.
[http://dx.doi.org/10.2217/nnm.15.95] [PMID: 26302331]

[142] Conde J, Tian F, Hernandez Y, *et al.* RNAi-based glyconanoparticles trigger apoptotic pathways for *in vitro* and *in vivo* enhanced cancer-cell killing. Nanoscale 2015; 7(19): 9083-91.
[http://dx.doi.org/10.1039/C4NR05742B] [PMID: 25924183]

[143] Bartel DP. MicroRNAs: genomics, biogenesis, mechanism, and function. Cell 2004; 116(2): 281-97.
[http://dx.doi.org/10.1016/S0092-8674(04)00045-5] [PMID: 14744438]

[144] Calin GA, Dumitru CD, Shimizu M, *et al.* Frequent deletions and down-regulation of micro- RNA genes miR15 and miR16 at 13q14 in chronic lymphocytic leukemia. Proc Natl Acad Sci USA 2002; 99(24): 15524-9.
[http://dx.doi.org/10.1073/pnas.242606799] [PMID: 12434020]

[145] Hatley ME, Patrick DM, Garcia MR, *et al.* Modulation of K-Ras-dependent lung tumorigenesis by MicroRNA-21. Cancer Cell 2010; 18(3): 282-93.
[http://dx.doi.org/10.1016/j.ccr.2010.08.013] [PMID: 20832755]

[146] Chen Y, Zhu X, Zhang X, Liu B, Huang L. Nanoparticles modified with tumor-targeting scFv deliver siRNA and miRNA for cancer therapy. Mol Ther 2010; 18(9): 1650-6.
[http://dx.doi.org/10.1038/mt.2010.136] [PMID: 20606648]

[147] Kim JH, Yeom JH, Ko JJ, *et al.* Effective delivery of anti-miRNA DNA oligonucleotides by functionalized gold nanoparticles. J Biotechnol 2011; 155(3): 287-92.
[http://dx.doi.org/10.1016/j.jbiotec.2011.07.014] [PMID: 21807040]

[148] Davidson BL, McCray PB Jr. Current prospects for RNA interference-based therapies. Nat Rev Genet 2011; 12(5): 329-40.
[http://dx.doi.org/10.1038/nrg2968] [PMID: 21499294]

[149] Yekta S, Shih IH, Bartel DP. MicroRNA-directed cleavage of HOXB8 mRNA. Science 2004; 304(5670): 594-6.
[http://dx.doi.org/10.1126/science.1097434] [PMID: 15105502]

[150] Farh KK, Grimson A, Jan C, *et al.* The widespread impact of mammalian MicroRNAs on mRNA repression and evolution. Science 2005; 310(5755): 1817-21.
[http://dx.doi.org/10.1126/science.1121158] [PMID: 16308420]

[151] Brennecke J, Stark A, Russell RB, Cohen SM. Principles of microRNA-target recognition. PLoS Biol 2005; 3(3): e85.
[http://dx.doi.org/10.1371/journal.pbio.0030085] [PMID: 15723116]

[152] McClorey G, Wood MJ. An overview of the clinical application of antisense oligonucleotides for

RNA-targeting therapies. Curr Opin Pharmacol 2015; 24: 52-8.
[http://dx.doi.org/10.1016/j.coph.2015.07.005] [PMID: 26277332]

[153] Geary RS, Norris D, Yu R, Bennett CF. Pharmacokinetics, biodistribution and cell uptake of antisense oligonucleotides. Adv Drug Deliv Rev 2015; 87: 46-51.
[http://dx.doi.org/10.1016/j.addr.2015.01.008] [PMID: 25666165]

[154] Chan JH, Lim S, Wong WS. Antisense oligonucleotides: from design to therapeutic application. Clin Exp Pharmacol Physiol 2006; 33(5-6): 533-40.
[http://dx.doi.org/10.1111/j.1440-1681.2006.04403.x] [PMID: 16700890]

[155] Crooke ST. Molecular mechanisms of action of antisense drugs. Biochim Biophys Acta 1999; 1489(1): 31-44.
[http://dx.doi.org/10.1016/S0167-4781(99)00148-7] [PMID: 10806995]

[156] Crooke ST. Progress in antisense technology: the end of the beginning. Methods Enzymol 2000; 313: 3-45.
[http://dx.doi.org/10.1016/S0076-6879(00)13003-4] [PMID: 10595347]

[157] Vinhas R, Fernandes AR, Baptista PV. Gold nanoparticles for BCR-ABL1 gene silencing: Improving tyrosine kinase inhibitor efficacy in chronic myeloid leukemia. Mol Ther Nucleic Acids 2017; 7: 408-16.
[http://dx.doi.org/10.1016/j.omtn.2017.05.003] [PMID: 28624216]

[158] Landen CN Jr, Chavez-Reyes A, Bucana C, *et al.* Therapeutic EphA2 gene targeting *in vivo* using neutral liposomal small interfering RNA delivery. Cancer Res 2005; 65(15): 6910-8.
[http://dx.doi.org/10.1158/0008-5472.CAN-05-0530] [PMID: 16061675]

[159] Semple SC, Akinc A, Chen J, *et al.* Rational design of cationic lipids for siRNA delivery. Nat Biotechnol 2010; 28(2): 172-6.
[http://dx.doi.org/10.1038/nbt.1602] [PMID: 20081866]

[160] Geisbert TW, Lee AC, Robbins M, *et al.* Postexposure protection of non-human primates against a lethal Ebola virus challenge with RNA interference: a proof-of-concept study. Lancet 2010; 375(9729): 1896-905.
[http://dx.doi.org/10.1016/S0140-6736(10)60357-1] [PMID: 20511019]

[161] Akinc A, Zumbuehl A, Goldberg M, *et al.* A combinatorial library of lipid-like materials for delivery of RNAi therapeutics. Nat Biotechnol 2008; 26(5): 561-9.
[http://dx.doi.org/10.1038/nbt1402] [PMID: 18438401]

[162] Love KT, Mahon KP, Levins CG, *et al.* Lipid-like materials for low-dose, *in vivo* gene silencing. Proc Natl Acad Sci USA 2010; 107(5): 1864-9.
[http://dx.doi.org/10.1073/pnas.0910603106] [PMID: 20080679]

[163] Gao S, Dagnaes-Hansen F, Nielsen EJ, *et al.* The effect of chemical modification and nanoparticle formulation on stability and biodistribution of siRNA in mice. Mol Ther 2009; 17(7): 1225-33.
[http://dx.doi.org/10.1038/mt.2009.91] [PMID: 19401674]

[164] McCarroll J, Baigude H, Yang CS, Rana TM. Nanotubes functionalized with lipids and natural amino acid dendrimers: a new strategy to create nanomaterials for delivering systemic RNAi. Bioconjug Chem 2010; 21(1): 56-63.
[http://dx.doi.org/10.1021/bc900296z] [PMID: 19957956]

[165] McNamara JO II, Andrechek ER, Wang Y, *et al.* Cell type-specific delivery of siRNAs with aptamer-siRNA chimeras. Nat Biotechnol 2006; 24(8): 1005-15.
[http://dx.doi.org/10.1038/nbt1223] [PMID: 16823371]

[166] Zhou J, Li H, Li S, Zaia J, Rossi JJ. Novel dual inhibitory function aptamer-siRNA delivery system for HIV-1 therapy. Mol Ther 2008; 16(8): 1481-9.
[http://dx.doi.org/10.1038/mt.2008.92] [PMID: 18461053]

[167] Suzuki K, Tsunekawa Y, Hernandez-Benitez R, *et al. In vivo* genome editing *via* CRISPR/Cas9

mediated homology-independent targeted integration. Nature 2016; 540(7631): 144-9.
[http://dx.doi.org/10.1038/nature20565] [PMID: 27851729]

[168] Merkert S, Martin U. Targeted genome engineering using designer nucleases: State of the art and practical guidance for application in human pluripotent stem cells. Stem Cell Res (Amst) 2016; 16(2): 377-86.
[http://dx.doi.org/10.1016/j.scr.2016.02.027] [PMID: 26921872]

[169] Carlson-Stevermer J, Abdeen AA, Kohlenberg L, *et al.* Assembly of CRISPR ribonucleoproteins with biotinylated oligonucleotides *via* an RNA aptamer for precise gene editing. Nat Commun 2017; 8(1): 1711.
[http://dx.doi.org/10.1038/s41467-017-01875-9] [PMID: 29167458]

[170] Liao HK, Hatanaka F, Araoka T, *et al. In vivo* target gene activation *via* CRISPR/Cas9-Mediated trans-epigenetic modulation. Cell 2017; 171(7): 1495-1507.e15.
[http://dx.doi.org/10.1016/j.cell.2017.10.025] [PMID: 29224783]

[171] Yin H, Song CQ, Dorkin JR, *et al.* Therapeutic genome editing by combined viral and non-viral delivery of CRISPR system components *in vivo*. Nat Biotechnol 2016; 34(3): 328-33.
[http://dx.doi.org/10.1038/nbt.3471] [PMID: 26829318]

[172] Mout R, Ray M, Lee YW, Scaletti F, Rotello VM. *In vivo* delivery of CRISPR/Cas9 for therapeutic gene editing: progress and challenges. Bioconjug Chem 2017; 28(4): 880-4.
[http://dx.doi.org/10.1021/acs.bioconjchem.7b00057] [PMID: 28263568]

[173] Peng R, Lin G, Li J. Potential pitfalls of CRISPR/Cas9-mediated genome editing. FEBS J 2016; 283(7): 1218-31.
[http://dx.doi.org/10.1111/febs.13586] [PMID: 26535798]

[174] Mitragotri S, Lammers T, Bae YH, *et al.* Drug delivery research for the future: expanding the nano horizons and beyond. J Control Release 2017; 246: 183-4.
[http://dx.doi.org/10.1016/j.jconrel.2017.01.011] [PMID: 28110715]

CHAPTER 5

Short Non-coding RNAs: Promising Biopharmaceutical Weapons in Breast Carcinogenesis

Rana Ahmed Youness[1,*] and **Mohamed Zakaria Gad**[2,*]

[1] *Pharmaceutical Biology Department, Faculty of Pharmacy and Biotechnology, German University in Cairo, New Cairo City, Main Entrance Al Tagamoa Al Khames, 11835, Cairo, Egypt*

[2] *Biochemistry Department, Faculty of Pharmacy and Biotechnology, German University in Cairo, New Cairo City, Main Entrance Al Tagamoa Al Khames, 11835, Cairo, Egypt*

Abstract: Despite being previously annotated as 'junk' transcriptional products, the non-coding RNA molecules (ncRNAs) have proven their indisputable role in carcinogenesis. ncRNAs are believed to act as potent oncogenic mediators or tumor suppressors in different contexts in oncology. Functionally, ncRNAs are able to modulate various processes in the cell such as chromatin re-modeling, transcription, post-transcriptional modifications and especially signal transduction. The most abundant and well-studied ncRNA molecules are the microRNAs (miRNAs/miRs). Different oncogenic signaling cascades have recently been in relation with miRNAs in a bi-directional crosstalk. Thus, this chapter offers a wider perspective towards complex networks of interactions coordinated by miRNAs specifically in Breast Cancer (BC). Nonetheless, this chapter also sheds the light onto clinical status of the miRNAs as a potential therapeutic intervention in several contexts.

Keywords: Breast Cancer, MicroRNAs, miR-34a, miR-21, MRX34, RG-012.

IN ONCOLOGY: IT IS NOT "ONE SIZE FITS ALL"

In-spite of the enormous efforts directed towards oncology research, its incidence rate and the number of cancer-related mortalities are still steeply rising [1], thus ringing a bell for a lot of limitations in the conventional therapeutic approaches and treatment protocols currently available for cancer patients. After decades of research and enormous observations, a new hypothesis is recently dominating the field of oncology which is "tumors are not alike". It has been recently stated that

* **Corresponding authors Dr. Rana Ahmed Youness:** Pharmaceutical Biology Department, Faculty of Pharmacy and Biotechnology, German University in Cairo, 11835, Cairo, Egypt; E-mails: rana.ahmed-youness@guc.edu.eg; rana.youness21@gmail.com, **Prof. Mohamed Zakaria Gad:** Biochemistry Department, Faculty of Pharmacy and Biotechnology, German University in Cairo, 11835, Cairo, Egypt; Tel: 002-01272222695; Fax: +202-2-2759 0711; E-mail: Mohamed.gad@guc.edu.eg

Yusuf Tutar (Ed.)

the heterogeneity among malignant tumors is refereed as one of the main obstacles leading to improper eradication of cancer until this moment [2].

Heterogeneity in solid tumors is classified into 3 main types: 1) inter-tumor heterogeneity among patients, 2) intra-tumor heterogeneity within the same tumor and 3) temporal heterogeneity in the tumor during developmental changes or changes in response to treatment [2], thus making the legend of cancer even more puzzling and challenging, and the introduction of "precision medicine" in oncology and its extrapolation to "personalized treatment code" for each cancer patient is a deep necessity.

Breast Cancer (BC)

Breast cancer (BC) comes on top of the list of such heterogeneous solid tumors. BC comprises a multiplicity of tumor subtypes that have various treatment responses since they are demonstrated in many clinical, pathological and molecular profiles [3]. It is also hypothesized that the reason many BC patients experience resistance to conventional protocols may be due to the heterogeneity of BC [4]. Furthermore, particular BC subtypes are described as being challenging and complicated in terms of diagnosis and treatment [3]. BC is the second most common malignancy in both sexes that comes after lung cancer, according to the "Globocan" project of the International Agency for Research on Cancer (IACR) [5]. Yet, it should be a research priority as it is the most common malignancy among females [5].

Incidence and Prevalence

Globally, BC comprises nearly 25% of all incident cancer cases [5]. BC is notoriously known for its high incidence rate in all countries [6]. According to the latest world cancer statistics available from the IARC around 1.7 million patients were diagnosed with BC and 577,000 women died in 2012 [5]. Almost 50% of BC patients are diagnosed in low- and middle-income countries, which is a disappointment because they are already experiencing a double burden of rising non-communicable diseases with existing prevalent infectious diseases [7]. Moreover, much higher mortality rates in these countries are seen considering the incidence-to-mortality ratio, with almost 60% of BC deaths [8]. It is also worth noting that a large variation has been observed in BC survival rates around the world, with an estimated 5-year survival rate that may reach to 80% in high income countries. However, less than 40% survival rate was experienced by patients in low income countries [9]. Such terrifying statistics are definitely suggesting slow progress made in the prevention setting of such dominating disease and the prominence of BC as an endemic tribulation in our countries.

BC is Not Just One Disease

Stemming from the unanimous heterogeneity of BC; BC is acknowledged for its disparate clinical behavior and patient outcomes [10]. Therefore, BC cannot be viewed as a single clinico-pathological entity, but it must be dissected into a number of more homogeneous entities known as BC subtypes. The idea that BC is not just a disease with a few variants, but a representative of diverse neoplastic diseases is also supported by the heterogeneity of BC among patients [11]. Distinct nature of such neoplastic diseases are usually realized through traditional pathological examination [12], however the actual great diversity among BC patients can be known only through molecular, proteomic and metabolic analyses as shown in Table **1** [13].

Table 1. Molecular Subtypes of BC.

Molecular Subtype	Biomarker Profile
Luminal A	ER^+ and/or PR^+, $HER\text{-}2^-$, and low Ki-67 (<14%)
Luminal B	ER^+ and/or PR^+ and $HER\text{-}2^+$ (luminal-HER2 group)
Luminal B-like	ER^+ and/or PR^+, $HER\text{-}2^-$, and high Ki-67 (≥14%)
HER-2	ER^-, PR^-, and $HER\text{-}2^+$
Triple Negative Breast Cancer (TNBC)	ER^-, PR^- and $HER\text{-}2^-$

Molecular Circuits Underlying BC

Heterogeneity concept in BC is also supported by molecular pathogenesis studies. BC was referred to as collection of diseases with variable molecular underpinnings modulating therapeutic responses, disease-free intervals, and long-term survival of patients [10]. It is very disappointing that the molecular basis of such malignant transformation process has remained elusive and considered as one of the most challenging aspects of the disease, given all current efforts directed towards research on BC [14]. Comprehensive analysis and assessment of the molecular features of the disorder is necessary to reach a true personalized BC treatment. Additionally, understanding the impact of specific genetic and epigenetic changes and their combinations is also necessary to achieve the goal of personalized management of patient [10]. Some molecular circuits that are changed are shown in Fig. (**1**) underlie in the pathogenesis of BC such as JAK/STAT, PI3K/AKT/mTOR and RAS/RAF/MAPK signaling pathways [15]. In this figure, oncogenic signaling cascades are drawn downstream from a collection of aberrantly expressed tyrosine kinase receptors (such as insulin like growth factor-1 receptor, IGF-1R), EGFR and HER-2 receptors or cytokines receptors (such as IL-1 and TNF-α), or chemokine receptors (such as C-C chemokine receptor type 7, CCR7 and C-X-C chemokine receptor type 4, CXCR4). BC is also known to be molecularly targeted by current drugs, as shown in Fig. (**1**), that block its oncogenic drivers such as Lapatinib inactivating EGFR and HER-2 receptors, Sorafenib blocking the RAS/RAF signaling cascade and Bortezomib blocking the activation of NF-κB. Though, a resistance mechanism was observed to develop against these drugs. Other parallel signaling pathways are usually activated following this resistance. Hence, when a single point in such convoluted circuits is targeted, this induces compensatory activation of an up- and/or down- stream corresponding oncogenic pathways which then result in drug resistance [16, 17]. A multi-functional player with the ability to repress multiple proteins rather than only one, and consequently shutting down deregulated pathways simultaneously would be very effective [18].

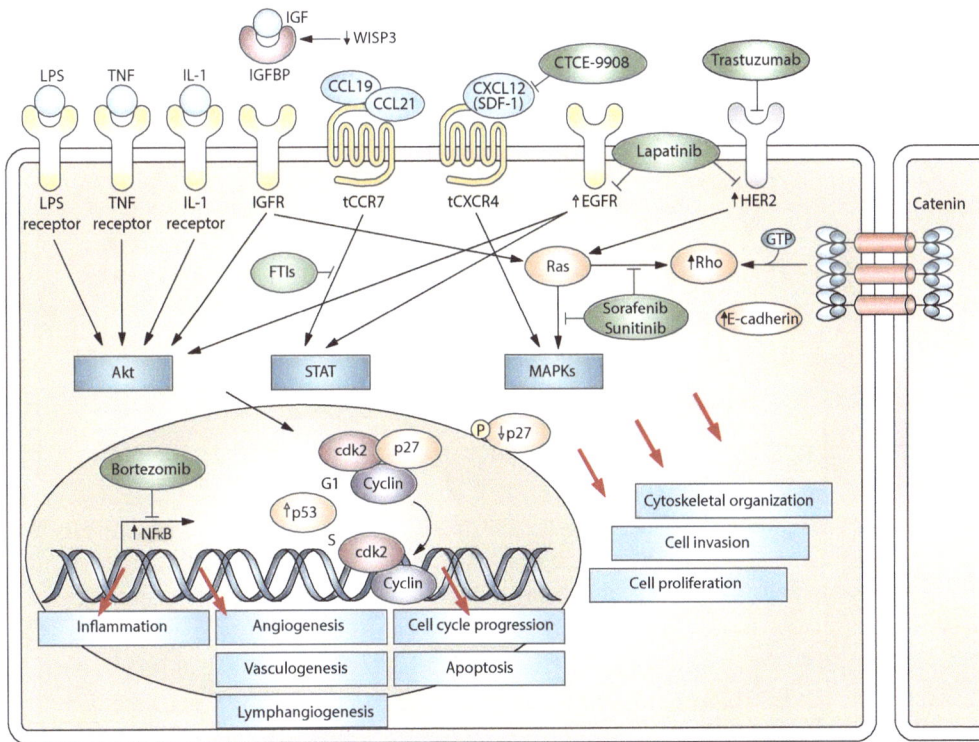

Fig. (1). Molecular signaling pathways orchestrating the high proliferative status of BC [15].

But the question now is: Is there a multi-functional upstream regulator capable of tuning more than one player in such inter-wined signaling cascades beginning with the receptors and their ligands ending with the oncogenic transcription factors?

These multi-functional tuners are endogenously expressed within our cells and are known as non-coding RNAs (ncRNAs). Therefore, the answer of this question is definitely "yes".

Non-coding RNAs (ncRNA)

Many specific ncRNA molecules have been identified in various cellular compartments [19]. According to earlier perceptions, ncRNAs were considered as 'junk' transcriptional products, but now they are known to be functional regulatory molecules. Several cellular processes such as; chromatin re-modeling, transcription, post-transcriptional modifications and most importantly signal transduction are potentially modulated by ncRNAs that have hundreds of targets that could simultaneously affect, thus nominating ncRNAs to play a key role in the process of carcinogenesis [19]. Small ncRNA molecules known as microRNAs (miRNAs/miRs) and the long ncRNA (lncRNA) molecules are the most abundant and well-studied ncRNAs. They have been identified as either oncogenic drivers or tumor suppressors in BC. Of note, ncRNAs have recently been involved in a bi-directional crosstalk among several oncogenic signaling cascades [20, 21]. In order to design better therapeutic interventions, interactions and complex networks coordinated by ncRNAs should be better understood [19].

MicroRNAs (miRNAs): Versatile Regulators of the Human Genome

As a class of small ncRNA molecules (~22 nucleotides (nt)), miRNAs can post-transcriptionally regulate almost 60% of human genome expression and thus are known to be the "Master-Maestro" of the genome [22, 23].

Biogenesis of miRNAs

The transcription process of miRNAs occurs in the nucleus by RNA polymerase II or III, and produces the primary miRNA (pri-miRNA), which possesses a 5'cap and a 3'-poly-A tail [24, 25]. This pri-miRNA is folded into one or more stem loop structures of approximately 30 bp flanked by two single stranded RNA (ssRNA) sequences at the base. In the nucleus, there are some RNA stem-loo--like structures which are distinguished from these primary transcripts with a unique ssRNA-dsRNA junction [26, 27]. DiGeorge syndrome critical region 8 (DGCR8) [26], which is a double stranded RNA-binding protein recognizing this characteristic junction and gives rise to a microprocessor complex in association with nuclear RNAase III ribonuclease, Drosha and additional proteins [28 - 30]. This complex cleaves the pri-miRNA stems mainly by means of the Drosharibonuclease activity, generating a 60-100 nt long hairpin precursor miRNA (pre-miRNA) with 5'-monophosphate and a 3'-2-nt overhang [31]. Exportin-5 (Exp-5) recognizes specific features in pre-miRNA [32, 33] then aids in its translocation from nucleus to cytoplasm in cooperation with guanine triphosphatase (GTPase) Ran [34]. In the cytoplasm, the pre-miRNA hairpin and the 3'-overhang are recognized by the cytoplasmic RNAse III ribonuclease, Dicer, which cleaves the loop and terminal base pairs of the pre-miRNA creating a ~22 ntmiRNA–miRNA* duplex having 2-nt 3'overhangs at both ends [35, 36]. In a similar pattern to the microprocessor complex in the nucleus, Dicer cleavage occurs in the cytoplasm in a larger complex including the human immunodeficiency virus trans-activating response RNA-binding protein (TRBP) that stabilizes the interaction of Dicer with pre-miRNA as its main function and contains three double stranded RNA-binding domains [37, 38]. After the cleavage process, an unidentified RNA helicase unwinds the miRNA duplex and the two strands are then separated into the "guide" strand, which is usually known as the mature miRNA, responsible for the post-transcriptional regulation of target mRNAs and its complementary "passenger" strand usually designated with an asterix (*) that it was known to be degraded [39]. However, recently it was found that this "passenger" strand is not always discarded, but may possess significant biological functions; such as cooperative regulation of type I interferon production in the case of miR-155 and miR-155* [40].

Only one miRNA strand of the duplex, whether the mature or the passenger, is loaded onto the argonaut protein (AGO) to form the programmed miRNA–RNA-induced silencing complex (miRISC). RISC consists of mainly Dicer, Ago proteins and other cellular components and is the final effector complex responsible for the executing the miRNA functions [37].

Mechanism of Action

miRISC complex formed at the end of the above mentioned processing steps is now able to bind to its target mRNA [41]. Target mRNA contains miRNA-binding sequence is generally referred to as the miRNA Recognitions Element (MRE) which pairs *via* nucleotide complementarity with the 6–8 nt stretch of the 5'-end of the miRNA known as the "seed sequence" [42, 43]. However, it is still not fully understood, how miRNAs find their intended targets [44], but it was suggested to be a diffusion driven process that also depends on the accessibility of the target sequence [45]. The mechanism by which the miRNA affects the mRNA depends on the degree of sequence complementarity and also on the nature of the specific Ago protein (which can be cleaving or non-cleaving) [45 - 47]. Most commonly, miRNAs negatively affect the translational process of their target mRNA, where the miRISC complex sterically hinder the ribosomal progression. In other cases, complete cleavage of the mRNA occurs and a reduction of the target mRNA as well as protein levels occur [48].

Involvement of miRNAs in BC Mystery

BC is a convoluted process as shown in Fig. (**1**). It involves tortuous molecular pathways and several factors, such as genetic mutations, abnormal expression of cellular proteins, inhibition of tumor suppressors, and overexpression of onco-genes. The recent evidence suggests that aberrant expression of key regulatory molecules such as miRNAs also massively contributes to the molecular pathophysiology of the disease [49]. miRNAs have been reported to be classified into two main classes; oncogenic miRNAs (tumor inducers), also known as oncomiRs. The second class is known as tumor suppressor miRNAs that usually target critical onco-proteins thus decreasing the tumor aggressiveness [49].

Oncogenic miRNAs (OncomiR) in BC

Aberrant expression of such oncomiRs in BC results is augmentation of the oncogenic signals and enhancing of cellular proliferation of BC cells [50]. Some potent tumor inducers miRNAs were found to be up-regulated, especially in BC with a high proliferation rates and cruel phenotypes such as TNBC [51]. Some of the oncomiRs aberrantly expressed in BC are listed in Table **2**. It is also important to note that some miRNAs play enhancing roles in the metastasis process, and recently known as "metasta-miRs" [52]. Such miRNAs were found to show more aggressive characteristics in promoting migration and invasiveness of tumor cells and they are usually correlated with poor prognosis of the disease. Some examples of such cantankerous metastamiRs in BC are listed in Table **2**.

Tumor Suppressor miRNAs in BC

Aggressiveness of BC could be attributed to miRNA down-regulation involved in tuning cell cycle, oncogenic signaling cascades and cellular apoptosis of BC cells. Some miRNAs that are annotated to act as tumor suppressor miRNAs in BC were found to be down-regulated and listed in Table **2**. Such tumor suppressor miRNAs were found to have pivotal roles in halting cancer progression through targeting critical onco-proteins such as *HER-2*, EGFR, IGF-1R and others restrain cell cycle progression through degrading several cell-cycle related proteins such as c-MYC and RB onco-proteins [18, 53 - 55]. Therefore, those miRNAs could be potentially used as a therapeutic tool for harnessing aggressive subtypes of BC.

Table 2. Examples of potential tumor-suppressor miRNAs, oncomiRs and metastamiRs in BC.

miRNA in BC	Tumor Suppressor miRNAs	Oncogenic miRNAs (OncomiRs)	Metastatic miRNAs (MetastamiRs)
hsa-miR-125	[56]		
hsa-miR-205	[57]		

(Table 2) cont.....

miRNA in BC	Tumor Suppressor miRNAs	Oncogenic miRNAs (OncomiRs)	Metastatic miRNAs (MetastamiRs)
hsa-miR-126	[53]		
hsa-miR-335	[53]		
hsa -miR-200c	[58]		
hsa-miR-127	[55]		
hsa-miR-17-5p	[59]		
hsa-miR-15/16	[53]		
hsa-miR-486-5p	[60]		
hsa-miR-497	[61]		
hsa-miR-196a		[62]	
hsa-miR-27a		[63]	
hsa-miR-106b		[64]	
hsa-miR-25		[64]	
hsa-miR-21		[65]	
hsa-miR-200a		[66]	
hsa-miR-221		[67]	
hsa-miR-155		[67]	
hsa-miR-182			[68]
hsa-miR-103			[69]
hsa-miR-132			[70]
hsa-miR-9			[71]
hsa-miR-374a			[72]
hsa-miR-210			[71]
hsa-miR-222			[73]

miRNAs as Potential Multi-targeted Therapeutic Tools

Within the last decade, a rapid progress has been witnessed in the field of miRNAs ranking them as crucial players in the malignant transformation process; this was based on strong validation analysis of some miRNAs and suggesting them as ideal candidates for therapeutic intervention [74]. With a role in hindering the antisense and siRNA therapeutics progress, successful pharmacological drug delivery has been the main focus of bringing miRNAs to cancer patients. Yet, miRNA therapeutics is considered within the realms of possibilities according to recent clinical success of current delivery technologies [74] and continuous emergence of new ones [74]. On the clinical translational level, great progress was witnessed in nominating several miRNAs to enter clinical trials after proving their potential roles in multiple cancers; however, until now, there is no potential miRNA was suggested to target BC and more specifically the aggressive phenotypes such as TNBC. Therefore, future research should be focused to find promising miRNAs and to increase their expressions in BC cells. At the same time future work can also focus on the finding of oncogenic miRNAs involved in TNBC and targeting them to stop tumor progression and metastasis [75].

A Brief Snapshot of Potential miRNAs Evading the Therapeutic Landscape

Currently, the translation process of miRNA based therapeutics from the bench to the clinic is guided by 4 leading RNA-therapeutic companies [76]. These companies have initiated and emerged an average of 20 clinical trials based on miRNAs and siRNAs. miRavirsen (a short Locked nucleic acid against miR-122) is the world's first miRNA-based therapeutic agent, which was developed by Santaris Pharma from Denmark to treat Hepatitis C virus (HCV) [77] and is the first miRNA-targeted drug to enter phase 2 clinical trials to unveil its safety profile and investigate its tolerability in HCV patients [76]. Nonetheless, several miRNAs can act as tumor suppressor genes as previously mentioned in this chapter including the well-known tumor suppressor miRNA, miR-34a [78]. miR-34a is usually de-regulated in several cancer patients including BC [78]. MRX34 is a miRNA-based pharmaceutical agent that delivers miR-34 mimics to perform its tumor suppressor activity in several cancers. Various cancers including colon cancer, non-small-cell lung cancer (NSCLC), hepatocellular carcinoma, cervical cancer, and ovarian cancer can use this drug. However, its clinical study was recently aborted in 2016 due to several severe adverse events (mainly immune-related side effects) [76]. Moreover, miR-21 was found to play an essential role in several fibrogenic diseases in several organs such as the kidneys [79]. Therefore, RG-012, antagomirs against miR-21 has been developed to prevent Alport nephropathy [80]. Alport syndrome is a deathly genetic kidney disease which currently lacks an approved therapy; however RG-012 is currently in the clinical trial pipeline for its treatment [80].

CONSENT FOR PUBLICATION

Not applicable.

CONFLICT OF INTEREST

The authors confirm that the contents of this chapter have no conflict of interest.

ACKNOWLEDGEMENTS

Declared none.

REFERENCES

[1]   Balogun OD, Formenti SC. Locally advanced breast cancer - strategies for developing nations. Front Oncol 2015; 5: 89.
        [http://dx.doi.org/10.3389/fonc.2015.00089] [PMID: 25964882]

[2]   Ellsworth RE, Blackburn HL, Shriver CD, Soon-Shiong P, Ellsworth DL. Molecular heterogeneity in breast cancer: State of the science and implications for patient care. Semin Cell Dev Biol 2017; 64: 65-72.
        [http://dx.doi.org/10.1016/j.semcdb.2016.08.025] [PMID: 27569190]

[3]   Yousef EM, Furrer D, Laperriere DL, *et al.* MCM2: An alternative to Ki-67 for measuring breast cancer cell proliferation. Mod Pathol 2017; 30(5): 682-97.
        [http://dx.doi.org/10.1038/modpathol.2016.231] [PMID: 28084344]

[4]   Turashvili G, Brogi E. Tumor Heterogeneity in Breast Cancer. Front Med (Lausanne) 2017; 4: 227.
        [http://dx.doi.org/10.3389/fmed.2017.00227] [PMID: 29276709]

[5]   Ferlay J, Soerjomataram I, Dikshit R, *et al.* Cancer incidence and mortality worldwide: sources, methods and major patterns in GLOBOCAN 2012. Int J Cancer 2015; 136(5): E359-86.
        [http://dx.doi.org/10.1002/ijc.29210] [PMID: 25220842]

[6]   Clegg LX, Reichman ME, Miller BA, *et al.* Impact of socioeconomic status on cancer incidence and stage at diagnosis: selected findings from the surveillance, epidemiology, and end results: National Longitudinal Mortality Study. Cancer Causes Control 2009; 20(4): 417-35.
        [http://dx.doi.org/10.1007/s10552-008-9256-0] [PMID: 19002764]

[7]   Harford JB. Breast-cancer early detection in low-income and middle-income countries: do what you can *versus* one size fits all. Lancet Oncol 2011; 12(3): 306-12.
        [http://dx.doi.org/10.1016/S1470-2045(10)70273-4] [PMID: 21376292]

[8]   Galukande M, Wabinga H, Mirembe F. Breast cancer survival experiences at a tertiary hospital in sub-Saharan Africa: a cohort study. World J Surg Oncol 2015; 13: 220.
        [http://dx.doi.org/10.1186/s12957-015-0632-4] [PMID: 26187151]

[9]   Coleman MP, Quaresma M, Berrino F, *et al.* Cancer survival in five continents: a worldwide population-based study (CONCORD). Lancet Oncol 2008; 9(8): 730-56.
        [http://dx.doi.org/10.1016/S1470-2045(08)70179-7] [PMID: 18639491]

[10]   Rivenbark AG, O'Connor SM, Coleman WB. Molecular and cellular heterogeneity in breast cancer: challenges for personalized medicine. Am J Pathol 2013; 183(4): 1113-24.
        [http://dx.doi.org/10.1016/j.ajpath.2013.08.002] [PMID: 23993780]

[11]   Polyak K. Breast cancer: origins and evolution. J Clin Invest 2007; 117(11): 3155-63.
        [http://dx.doi.org/10.1172/JCI33295] [PMID: 17975657]

[12]   Rosen PP. The pathological classification of human mammary carcinoma: past, present and future. Ann Clin Lab Sci 1979; 9(2): 144-56.
        [PMID: 453788]

[13]   Koboldt DC. Cancer Genome Atlas Network. Comprehensive molecular portraits of human breast tumours. Nature 2012; 490(7418): 61-70.
        [http://dx.doi.org/10.1038/nature11412] [PMID: 23000897]

[14]   Jemal A, Siegel R, Ward E, *et al.* Cancer statistics, 2006. CA Cancer J Clin 2006; 56(2): 106-30.
        [http://dx.doi.org/10.3322/canjclin.56.2.106] [PMID: 16514137]

[15]   Yamauchi H, Cristofanilli M, Nakamura S, Hortobagyi GN, Ueno NT. Molecular targets for treatment

of inflammatory breast cancer. Nat Rev Clin Oncol 2009; 6(7): 387-94.
[http://dx.doi.org/10.1038/nrclinonc.2009.73] [PMID: 19468291]

[16]   O'Reilly KE, Rojo F, She QB, *et al.* mTOR inhibition induces upstream receptor tyrosine kinase signaling and activates Akt. Cancer Res 2006; 66(3): 1500-8.
[http://dx.doi.org/10.1158/0008-5472.CAN-05-2925] [PMID: 16452206]

[17]   Zitzmann K, Rüden Jv, Brand S, *et al.* Compensatory activation of Akt in response to mTOR and Raf inhibitors - a rationale for dual-targeted therapy approaches in neuroendocrine tumor disease. Cancer Lett 2010; 295(1): 100-9.
[http://dx.doi.org/10.1016/j.canlet.2010.02.018] [PMID: 20356670]

[18]   Youness RA, El-Tayebi HM, Assal RA, Hosny K, Esmat G, Abdelaziz AI. MicroRNA-486-5p enhances hepatocellular carcinoma tumor suppression through repression of IGF-1R and its downstream mTOR, STAT3 and c-Myc. Oncol Lett 2016; 12(4): 2567-73.
[http://dx.doi.org/10.3892/ol.2016.4914] [PMID: 27698829]

[19]   Anastasiadou E, Jacob LS, Slack FJ. Non-coding RNA networks in cancer. Nat Rev Cancer 2018; 18(1): 5-18.
[http://dx.doi.org/10.1038/nrc.2017.99] [PMID: 29170536]

[20]   Zhai Y, Tyagi SC, Tyagi N. Cross-talk of MicroRNA and hydrogen sulfide: A novel therapeutic approach for bone diseases. Biomed Pharmacother 2017; 92: 1073-84.
[http://dx.doi.org/10.1016/j.biopha.2017.06.007] [PMID: 28618652]

[21]   Hackfort BT, Mishra PK. Emerging role of hydrogen sulfide-microRNA crosstalk in cardiovascular diseases. Am J Physiol Heart Circ Physiol 2016; 310(7): H802-12.
[http://dx.doi.org/10.1152/ajpheart.00660.2015] [PMID: 26801305]

[22]   Espinoza-Lewis RA, Wang DZ. MicroRNAs in heart development. Curr Top Dev Biol 2012; 100: 279-317.
[http://dx.doi.org/10.1016/B978-0-12-387786-4.00009-9] [PMID: 22449848]

[23]   Friedman RC, Farh KK, Burge CB, Bartel DP. Most mammalian mRNAs are conserved targets of microRNAs. Genome Res 2009; 19(1): 92-105.
[http://dx.doi.org/10.1101/gr.082701.108] [PMID: 18955434]

[24]   Borchert GM, Lanier W, Davidson BL. RNA polymerase III transcribes human microRNAs. Nat Struct Mol Biol 2006; 13(12): 1097-101.
[http://dx.doi.org/10.1038/nsmb1167] [PMID: 17099701]

[25]   Denli AM, Tops BB, Plasterk RH, Ketting RF, Hannon GJ. Processing of primary microRNAs by the Microprocessor complex. Nature 2004; 432(7014): 231-5.
[http://dx.doi.org/10.1038/nature03049] [PMID: 15531879]

[26]   Han J, Lee Y, Yeom KH, *et al.* Molecular basis for the recognition of primary microRNAs by the Drosha-DGCR8 complex. Cell 2006; 125(5): 887-901.
[http://dx.doi.org/10.1016/j.cell.2006.03.043] [PMID: 16751099]

[27]   Zeng Y, Cullen BR. Efficient processing of primary microRNA hairpins by Drosha requires flanking nonstructured RNA sequences. J Biol Chem 2005; 280(30): 27595-603.
[http://dx.doi.org/10.1074/jbc.M504714200] [PMID: 15932881]

[28]   Gregory RI, Yan KP, Amuthan G, *et al.* The Microprocessor complex mediates the genesis of microRNAs. Nature 2004; 432(7014): 235-40.
[http://dx.doi.org/10.1038/nature03120] [PMID: 15531877]

[29]   Han J, Lee Y, Yeom KH, Kim YK, Jin H, Kim VN. The Drosha-DGCR8 complex in primary microRNA processing. Genes Dev 2004; 18(24): 3016-27.
[http://dx.doi.org/10.1101/gad.1262504] [PMID: 15574589]

[30]   Lee Y, Ahn C, Han J, *et al.* The nuclear RNase III Drosha initiates microRNA processing. Nature 2003; 425(6956): 415-9.

[http://dx.doi.org/10.1038/nature01957] [PMID: 14508493]

[31]   Basyuk E, Suavet F, Doglio A, Bordonné R, Bertrand E. Human let-7 stem-loop precursors harbor features of RNase III cleavage products. Nucleic Acids Res 2003; 31(22): 6593-7.
[http://dx.doi.org/10.1093/nar/gkg855] [PMID: 14602919]

[32]   Lund E, Güttinger S, Calado A, Dahlberg JE, Kutay U. Nuclear export of microRNA precursors. Science 2004; 303(5654): 95-8.
[http://dx.doi.org/10.1126/science.1090599] [PMID: 14631048]

[33]   Yi R, Qin Y, Macara IG, Cullen BR. Exportin-5 mediates the nuclear export of pre-microRNAs and short hairpin RNAs. Genes Dev 2003; 17(24): 3011-6.
[http://dx.doi.org/10.1101/gad.1158803] [PMID: 14681208]

[34]   Bohnsack MT, Czaplinski K, Gorlich D. Exportin 5 is a RanGTP-dependent dsRNA-binding protein that mediates nuclear export of pre-miRNAs. RNA 2004; 10(2): 185-91.
[http://dx.doi.org/10.1261/rna.5167604] [PMID: 14730017]

[35]   Bernstein E, Caudy AA, Hammond SM, Hannon GJ. Role for a bidentate ribonuclease in the initiation step of RNA interference. Nature 2001; 409(6818): 363-6.
[http://dx.doi.org/10.1038/35053110] [PMID: 11201747]

[36]   Hutvágner G, McLachlan J, Pasquinelli AE, Bálint E, Tuschl T, Zamore PD. A cellular function for the RNA-interference enzyme Dicer in the maturation of the let-7 small temporal RNA. Science 2001; 293(5531): 834-8.
[http://dx.doi.org/10.1126/science.1062961] [PMID: 11452083]

[37]   Chendrimada TP, Gregory RI, Kumaraswamy E, *et al.* TRBP recruits the Dicer complex to Ago2 for microRNA processing and gene silencing. Nature 2005; 436(7051): 740-4.
[http://dx.doi.org/10.1038/nature03868] [PMID: 15973356]

[38]   Förstemann K, Tomari Y, Du T, *et al.* Normal microRNA maturation and germ-line stem cell maintenance requires Loquacious, a double-stranded RNA-binding domain protein. PLoS Biol 2005; 3(7): e236.
[http://dx.doi.org/10.1371/journal.pbio.0030236] [PMID: 15918770]

[39]   Lau NC, Lim LP, Weinstein EG, Bartel DP. An abundant class of tiny RNAs with probable regulatory roles in Caenorhabditis elegans. Science 2001; 294(5543): 858-62.
[http://dx.doi.org/10.1126/science.1065062] [PMID: 11679671]

[40]   Zhou H, Huang X, Cui H, *et al.* miR-155 and its star-form partner miR-155* cooperatively regulate type I interferon production by human plasmacytoid dendritic cells. Blood 2010; 116(26): 5885-94.
[http://dx.doi.org/10.1182/blood-2010-04-280156] [PMID: 20852130]

[41]   Lages E, Ipas H, Guttin A, Nesr H, Berger F, Issartel JP. MicroRNAs: molecular features and role in cancer. Front Biosci 2012; 17: 2508-40.
[http://dx.doi.org/10.2741/4068] [PMID: 22652795]

[42]   Shukla GC, Singh J, Barik S. MicroRNAs: Processing, maturation, target recognition and regulatory functions. Mol Cell Pharmacol 2011; 3(3): 83-92.
[PMID: 22468167]

[43]   Winter J, Jung S, Keller S, Gregory RI, Diederichs S. Many roads to maturity: microRNA biogenesis pathways and their regulation. Nat Cell Biol 2009; 11(3): 228-34.
[http://dx.doi.org/10.1038/ncb0309-228] [PMID: 19255566]

[44]   Bartel DP. MicroRNAs: target recognition and regulatory functions. Cell 2009; 136(2): 215-33.
[http://dx.doi.org/10.1016/j.cell.2009.01.002] [PMID: 19167326]

[45]   Ameres SL, Martinez J, Schroeder R. Molecular basis for target RNA recognition and cleavage by human RISC. Cell 2007; 130(1): 101-12.
[http://dx.doi.org/10.1016/j.cell.2007.04.037] [PMID: 17632058]

[46]   Brennecke J, Stark A, Russell RB, Cohen SM. Principles of microRNA-target recognition. PLoS Biol 2005; 3(3): e85.
[http://dx.doi.org/10.1371/journal.pbio.0030085] [PMID: 15723116]

[47]   Witkos TM, Koscianska E, Krzyzosiak WJ. Practical aspects of microRNA target prediction. Curr Mol Med 2011; 11(2): 93-109.
[http://dx.doi.org/10.2174/156652411794859250] [PMID: 21342132]

[48]   Hutvágner G, Zamore PD. A microRNA in a multiple-turnover RNAi enzyme complex. Science 2002; 297(5589): 2056-60.
[http://dx.doi.org/10.1126/science.1073827] [PMID: 12154197]

[49]   Croce CM. Causes and consequences of microRNA dysregulation in cancer. Nat Rev Genet 2009; 10(10): 704-14.
[http://dx.doi.org/10.1038/nrg2634] [PMID: 19763153]

[50]   Sun J, Lu H, Wang X, Jin H. MicroRNAs in hepatocellular carcinoma: regulation, function, and clinical implications. Sci World J 2013; 2013: : 924206..
[http://dx.doi.org/10.1155/2013/924206] [PMID: 23431261]

[51]   Koleckova M, Janikova M, Kolar Z. MicroRNAs in triple-negative breast cancer. Neoplasma 2018; 65(1): 1-13.
[http://dx.doi.org/10.4149/neo_2018_170115N36] [PMID: 29322783]

[52]   Mehrgou A, Akouchekian M. Therapeutic impacts of microRNAs in breast cancer by their roles in regulating processes involved in this disease. J Res Med Sci 2017; 22: 130.
[http://dx.doi.org/10.4103/jrms.JRMS_967_16] [PMID: 29387117]

[53]   Tavazoie SF, Alarcón C, Oskarsson T, *et al.* Endogenous human microRNAs that suppress breast cancer metastasis. Nature 2008; 451(7175): 147-52.
[http://dx.doi.org/10.1038/nature06487] [PMID: 18185580]

[54]   Scott GK, Goga A, Bhaumik D, Berger CE, Sullivan CS, Benz CC. Coordinate suppression of ERBB2 and ERBB3 by enforced expression of micro-RNA miR-125a or miR-125b. J Biol Chem 2007; 282(2): 1479-86.
[http://dx.doi.org/10.1074/jbc.M609383200] [PMID: 17110380]

[55]   Saito Y, Liang G, Egger G, *et al.* Specific activation of microRNA-127 with downregulation of the proto-oncogene BCL6 by chromatin-modifying drugs in human cancer cells. Cancer Cell 2006; 9(6): 435-43.
[http://dx.doi.org/10.1016/j.ccr.2006.04.020] [PMID: 16766263]

[56]   Zhang Y, Yan LX, Wu QN, *et al.* miR-125b is methylated and functions as a tumor suppressor by regulating the ETS1 proto-oncogene in human invasive breast cancer. Cancer Res 2011; 71(10): 3552-62.
[http://dx.doi.org/10.1158/0008-5472.CAN-10-2435] [PMID: 21444677]

[57]   Joerger AC, Fersht AR. Structure-function-rescue: the diverse nature of common p53 cancer mutants. Oncogene 2007; 26(15): 2226-42.
[http://dx.doi.org/10.1038/sj.onc.1210291] [PMID: 17401432]

[58]   Ren Y, Han X, Yu K, *et al.* microRNA-200c downregulates XIAP expression to suppress proliferation and promote apoptosis of triple-negative breast cancer cells. Mol Med Rep 2014; 10(1): 315-21.
[http://dx.doi.org/10.3892/mmr.2014.2222] [PMID: 24821285]

[59]   Hossain A, Kuo MT, Saunders GF. Mir-17-5p regulates breast cancer cell proliferation by inhibiting translation of AIB1 mRNA. Mol Cell Biol 2006; 26(21): 8191-201.
[http://dx.doi.org/10.1128/MCB.00242-06] [PMID: 16940181]

[60]   Zhang G, Liu Z, Cui G, Wang X, Yang Z. MicroRNA-486-5p targeting PIM-1 suppresses cell proliferation in breast cancer cells. Tumour Biol 2014; 35(11): 11137-45.
[http://dx.doi.org/10.1007/s13277-014-2412-0] [PMID: 25104088]

[61]   Luo Q, Li X, Gao Y, *et al.* MiRNA-497 regulates cell growth and invasion by targeting cyclin E1 in breast cancer. Cancer Cell Int 2013; 13(1): 95.
[http://dx.doi.org/10.1186/1475-2867-13-95] [PMID: 24112607]

[62]   Luthra R, Singh RR, Luthra MG, *et al.* MicroRNA-196a targets annexin A1: a microRNA-mediated mechanism of annexin A1 downregulation in cancers. Oncogene 2008; 27(52): 6667-78.
[http://dx.doi.org/10.1038/onc.2008.256] [PMID: 18663355]

[63]   Mertens-Talcott SU, Chintharlapalli S, Li X, Safe S. The oncogenic microRNA-27a targets genes that regulate specificity protein transcription factors and the G2-M checkpoint in MDA-MB-231 breast cancer cells. Cancer Res 2007; 67(22): 11001-11.
[http://dx.doi.org/10.1158/0008-5472.CAN-07-2416] [PMID: 18006846]

[64]   Ivanovska I, Ball AS, Diaz RL, *et al.* MicroRNAs in the miR-106b family regulate p21/CDKN1A and promote cell cycle progression. Mol Cell Biol 2008; 28(7): 2167-74.
[http://dx.doi.org/10.1128/MCB.01977-07] [PMID: 18212054]

[65]   Huang GL, Zhang XH, Guo GL, *et al.* Clinical significance of miR-21 expression in breast cancer: SYBR-Green I-based real-time RT-PCR study of invasive ductal carcinoma. Oncol Rep 2009; 21(3): 673-9.
[PMID: 19212625]

[66]   Yu SJ, Hu JY, Kuang XY, *et al.* MicroRNA-200a promotes anoikis resistance and metastasis by targeting YAP1 in human breast cancer. Clin Cancer Res 2013; 19(6): 1389-99.
[http://dx.doi.org/10.1158/1078-0432.CCR-12-1959] [PMID: 23340296]

[67]   Deng L, Lei Q, Wang Y, *et al.* Downregulation of miR-221-3p and upregulation of its target gene PARP1 are prognostic biomarkers for triple negative breast cancer patients and associated with poor prognosis. Oncotarget 2017; 8(65): 108712-25.
[http://dx.doi.org/10.18632/oncotarget.21561] [PMID: 29312562]

[68]   Guttilla IK, White BA. Coordinate regulation of FOXO1 by miR-27a, miR-96, and miR-182 in breast cancer cells. J Biol Chem 2009; 284(35): 23204-16.
[http://dx.doi.org/10.1074/jbc.M109.031427] [PMID: 19574223]

[69]   Martello G, Rosato A, Ferrari F, *et al.* A MicroRNA targeting dicer for metastasis control. Cell 2010; 141(7): 1195-207.
[http://dx.doi.org/10.1016/j.cell.2010.05.017] [PMID: 20603000]

[70]   Anand S, Majeti BK, Acevedo LM, *et al.* MicroRNA-132-mediated loss of p120RasGAP activates the endothelium to facilitate pathological angiogenesis. Nat Med 2010; 16(8): 909-14.
[http://dx.doi.org/10.1038/nm.2186] [PMID: 20676106]

[71]   Iorio MV, Ferracin M, Liu CG, *et al.* MicroRNA gene expression deregulation in human breast cancer. Cancer Res 2005; 65(16): 7065-70.
[http://dx.doi.org/10.1158/0008-5472.CAN-05-1783] [PMID: 16103053]

[72]   Cai J, Guan H, Fang L, *et al.* MicroRNA-374a activates Wnt/β-catenin signaling to promote breast cancer metastasis. J Clin Invest 2013; 123(2): 566-79.
[http://dx.doi.org/10.1172/JCI65871] [PMID: 23321667]

[73]   Stinson S, Lackner MR, Adai AT, *et al.* TRPS1 targeting by miR-221/222 promotes the epithelial-t--mesenchymal transition in breast cancer. Sci Signal 2011; 4: 41.

[74]   Bader AG, Brown D, Stoudemire J, Lammers P. Developing therapeutic microRNAs for cancer. Gene Ther 2011; 18(12): 1121-6.
[http://dx.doi.org/10.1038/gt.2011.79] [PMID: 21633392]

[75]   D'Ippolito E, Iorio MV. MicroRNAs and triple negative breast cancer. Int J Mol Sci 2013; 14(11): 22202-20.
[http://dx.doi.org/10.3390/ijms141122202] [PMID: 24284394]

[76]   Chakraborty C, Sharma AR, Sharma G, Doss CGP, Lee SS. Therapeutic miRNA and siRNA: Moving from Bench to Clinic as Next Generation Medicine. Mol Ther Nucleic Acids 2017; 8: 132-43.
[http://dx.doi.org/10.1016/j.omtn.2017.06.005] [PMID: 28918016]

[77]   Lindow M, Kauppinen S. Discovering the first microRNA-targeted drug. J Cell Biol 2012; 199(3): 407-12.
[http://dx.doi.org/10.1083/jcb.201208082] [PMID: 23109665]

[78]   Bouchie A. First microRNA mimic enters clinic. Nat Biotechnol 2013; 31(7): 577.
[http://dx.doi.org/10.1038/nbt0713-577] [PMID: 23839128]

[79]   Chau BN, Xin C, Hartner J, *et al.* MicroRNA-21 promotes fibrosis of the kidney by silencing metabolic pathways. Sci Transl Med 2012; 4(121): : 121ra18..
[http://dx.doi.org/10.1126/scitranslmed.3003205] [PMID: 22344686]

[80]   Gomez IG, MacKenna DA, Johnson BG, *et al.* Anti-microRNA-21 oligonucleotides prevent Alport nephropathy progression by stimulating metabolic pathways. J Clin Invest 2015; 125(1): 141-56.
[http://dx.doi.org/10.1172/JCI75852] [PMID: 25415439]

CHAPTER 6

Combining Imaging and Drug Delivery for Cancer Treatment

Seda Keleştemur[1,*] and Gamze Yeşilay[2]

[1] *Department of Biotechnology, University of Health Sciences-Turkey, Hamidiye Institue of Health Sciences, Selimiye Mah., 34668, Istanbul, Turkey*

[2] *Department of Molecular Biology and Genetics, University of Health Sciences-Turkey, Hamidiye Health Sciences Institue, Selimiye Mah., 34668, Istanbul, Turkey*

Abstract: Theranostics is the definition of bringing the imaging agent and therapeutic drug together in the same delivery design. The term 'theranostic' was first defined by John Funkhouser in 2002 and since then it became one of the most attractive fields in treatment of severe diseases. Nanoparticles (NPs) are the most suitable carrier systems due to their plasmonic and magnetic properties, active surface areas and various physicochemical properties. Development of therapeutic NPs provide both active and passive targeting, sensitive monitoring of biological circulation, effective drug carrying and releasing, longer circulation time and efficient clearance from renal system. Here in this chapter, we discussed commonly used cancer treatment theranostic NPs that utilize imaging modalities such as magnetic resonance imaging (MRI), radionuclide-based imaging; positron emission tomography (PET) and single-photon emission computed tomography (SPECT) and X-ray-computed tomography (CT).

Keywords: Cancer, Computed tomography, Drug delivery, Imaging, Magnetic resonance imaging, Nanoparticles, Radionuclide-based imaging, Theranostic.

INTRODUCTION

The importance of diagnosis in the treatment of severe diseases and especially in cancers is high. Therefore, efforts are accumulated on the development of smarter diagnostic systems.

An emerging branch of diagnostic approaches is the design of theranostic particles where both 'thera'py and diag'nostics' is made possible with one particle. In classical diagnosis, if we take magnetic resonance imaging as an example, a high concentration of contrast agent is given to patient to obtain higher sensitivity. By utilizing theranostics, it is aimed to deliver a therapeutic dose while the patient al-

---

* **Corresponding author Seda Keleştemur:** Department of Biotechnology, University of Health Sciences-Turkey, Hamidiye Institue of Health Sciences, Selimiye Mah., 34668, Istanbul, Turkey; E-mail: seda.kelestemur@sbu.edu.tr

Yusuf Tutar (Ed.)

ready received high amount of exogenous material and while a high spatial resolution is obtained to monitor the disease region.

Nanomaterials are a promising platform to design smart theranostic tools for their biocompatible size range, modifiable surface, high surface-to-volume ratio that can enable higher drug loading efficiency, and excellent optical and electrical properties that can enable tunable photodynamic therapy (PDT), photothermal therapy (PTT) and many other possible modalities.

Here in this chapter, it was aimed to introduce nanotheranostic approaches in the treatment of cancers by grouping into imaging modalities. Under each imaging modality, innovative nanoparticle (NP) designs were explained and examples from the recent literature were provided.

Magnetic Resonance Imaging

Magnetic resonance imaging (MRI) is a valuable tool in soft tissue imaging together with its high spatial resolution and tissue depth-independent imaging abilities. Utilization of tissue contrasting agents provides extra sensitivity to the technique. Moreover, by modifying the contrast agents, theranostic applications of MRI is made possible alongside with tracking the payload release by measuring changes in T_1 and T_2 relaxation, and chemical exchange saturation transition (CEST) contrast in tissue of interest [1 - 3].

Current theranostic MRI applications mostly include; pH- [4, 5], hyperthermia- [6], light- [7] or ultrasound-mediated [8] chemotherapeutic drug release, PDT [9 - 11] or PTT [12, 13], siRNA-mediated gene knockdown [13, 14], microbubble generation upon laser irradiation [15] or ultrasound stimulus [8] as well as magnet-guided tissue localization of liposomes [16].

The drug and contrasting agent carrier systems can also be coated with various materials. Coating enables targeted delivery of drugs by the help of targeting moieties such as anti-EGFR [17], anti-VEGF [18], aptamers [4] or folate [19], depending on the tissue or tumor of interest. Polyethylene glycol (PEG) can be used to enhance biocompatibility of metals such as Gd^{3+}, which is used as contrasting agent for MRI [20, 21]. It is possible to increase drug-loading capacity by utilizing polymers to load contrasting agents on them [13] or to cross challenging barriers in the body such as blood-brain-barrier (BBB) by utilizing surfactants such as Tween-20 [22].

There are several approaches to obtain a final theranostic agent for MRI applications. For instance, NPs such as SPIONs are used as contrast agents and can be loaded in liposomes together with a chemotherapeutic drug [22]. Once they reach tumor site, the drug is released whereas tissue contrast is obtained in MRI.

Liposomal delivery is actually widely investigated strategy for its ability to deliver large payloads at once. Various compositions of liposomes enable more efficient cargo delivery to the tissue of interest. Among them, long-circulating liposomes, which are mostly coated with a stealth polymer such as PEG, are promising theranostic tools. These sterically stabilized liposomes provide escape from reticuloendothelial system (RES) and increase tumor accumulation [23]. Addition of a targeting moiety to the liposome increases the tumor accumulation and minimizes non-specific tissue damage. For instance, in a study by Kwon *et al.,* anti-EGFR antibody was coated on liposome surface where the MagLipo liposomes contained magnetic iron oxide NP core-SiO_2 shell [17]. The liposomes were also loaded with doxorubicin (Dox) as a chemotherapeutic drug and siRNA against Plk1, a gene overexpressed in pancreas cancer. These pH-sensitive liposomes showed successful therapeutic effect *in vitro*. Another interesting liposomal nanotheranostic tool is self-assembling ABCD NPs. The ABCD NP concept was introduced by Kostarelos and Miller in 2005 [24], where each layer was named after each letters of ABCD. The core layer (layer A) is a nucleic acid layer such as siRNA, mRNA, or pDNA. Then comes layers B, C, and D corresponding to lipid envelope layer, stealth or biocompatibility layer, and biological recognition layer, respectively. They also suggested that NPs containing only AB layers can be used *in vitro*, whereas ABCD or ABC NPs can be utilized *in vivo*. An application of this approach can be exemplified from a study by Kenny *et al.* [14], where they designed a nanotheranostic agent against ovarian cancer on OVCAR-3 human ovarian cancer xenograft mice and they termed the particles as liposome-entrapped siRNA (LEsiRNA). The particles contained anti-Survivin siRNA entrapped in pegylated cationic liposomes and the liposome formulation contained Rhodamine and Gd-DOTA which provided bimodal imaging; fluorescent and MRI, respectively. In a similar approach, Liu *et al.* designed a multilayered particle [25]. In the core layer, there were Fe_3O_4 NPs whereas a mesoporous SiO_2 layer covered this layer to form magnetic mesoporous silica NPs (FM). The porous structure of FM was doped with Dox and the particles were entrapped in a lipid bilayer, which was loaded with zinc phtalocyanine for PDT. Finally, the bilayer was coated with PEG-Methotrexate for chemotherapeutic effect. All of these modifications provided magnet-guided localization, stimuli and pH-triggered release of drugs whereas trimodal imaging was made possible; MRI, fluorescent and photoacoustic imaging.

Polymers have been applied as drug and contrast agent carriers. Among others, poly(lactic-co-glycolic acid) (PLGA)-based systems have been widely tested *in vivo* for the theranostics of various cancers in animal models. In many cases, the polymer is loaded with perfluorocarbon or perfluorohexane gas together with a chemotherapeutic drug such as Dox. Once the agents are injected into the tested animal systems, either high- or low-intensity focused ultrasound is applied to initiate microbubble formation to enhance therapeutic effect by tumor ablation together with enhanced contrast in ultrasound imaging. Moreover, the ultrasound stimulus initiates drug release from the polymer [26, 27]. Instead of embedding drugs and contrasting agents into polymers, another approach is to coat them on magnetic NPs, which then increases biocompatibility of the particles. For instance, in a study by Mrowczynski *et al.*, a polydopamine (PDA) shell was applied on Fe_3O_4 core NPs [28]. To improve drug-loading efficiency, PDA shell was coated with beta-cyclodextrins loaded with hydrophobic drug, Dox. In another study, dopamine was polymerized together with Dox on $CoFe_2O_4$ core NPs to form a PDA layer [16] (Fig. **1**). The surface was coated with ZIF-8, a metal-organic-framework (MOF), whereas the hydrophobic chemotherapeutic drug campthotecin was encapsulated between the PDA and ZIF-8. With this strategy, a two-step release of chemotherapeutic drugs was aimed and a fast release of drugs was achieved at tumor site, whereas PTT enhanced therapeutic efficiency. An additional magnetic field provided targeted MRI.

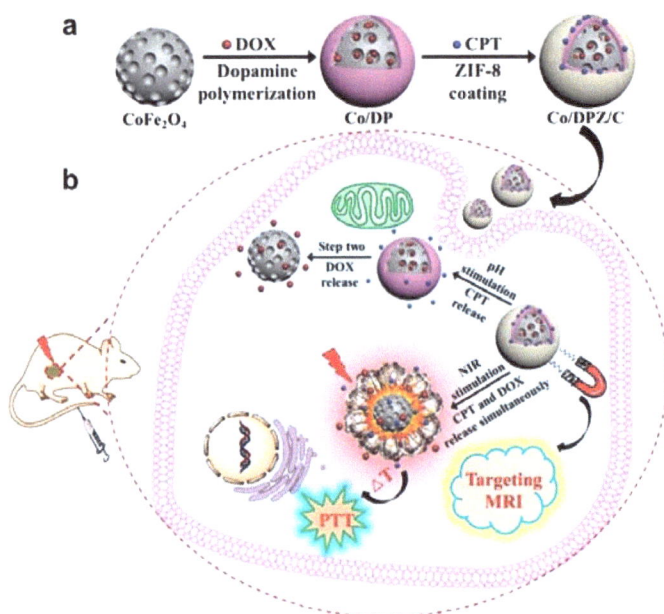

Fig. (1). (a) Synthesis of PDA coated $CoFe_2O_4$ nanocarrier (b) theranostic strategy of the nanocarrier for MRI-guided multi-drug chemotherapy and PTT synergistic therapy with pH and NIR-stimulation release. (DOX: doxorubicin, CPT: campthotecin, Co/DPZ/C: overall name of the synthesized nanocarrier) Reprinted with permission from (Yang *et al.*, 2017) [16]. Copyright 2017 American Chemical Society.

In the above-mentioned study, the nanocarrier is actually classified as a nanocomposite. Nanocomposites have also become an attractive field of investigation in nanotheranostics to be applied in MRI. Various cores such as polypyrrole and Prussian blue can be coupled with a MOF shell such as MIL-100-Fe and loaded with Dox or a drug with lower toxicity such as artemisinin to provide chemophotothermal therapy coupled with pH-triggered drug release [29]. Depending on the core structure, bimodal imaging can be achieved. For instance, a polypyrrole core enables photoacoustic imaging, whereas the Prussian blue core enables fluorescent imaging in addition to MRI.

Various other examples of smart-designs are gaining attention for MRI nanotheranostics applications. For instance, graphene oxide sheets were chosen for their greater biocompatibility, and stability in aqueous solutions [30]. 2D-layered double hydroxides with Cu were loaded with drug 5-FU to obtain a synergistic NIR PTT and chemotherapeutic effect [31]. As a stealth layer to escape from RES, use of hepatitis B virus core protein (HBc) shell on Fe_3O_4 NPs modified with methotrexate was reported [32]. The obtained virus like particles were more efficiently uptaken by the tumor cells of BALB/c mice injected with 4T1 breast cancer cells. Another drug release approach is to make use of increased thiols in tumor environment to break S-S bonds of Dox conjugates as reported by Lee *et al.* [21]. To the bilayer of liposome, Gd^{3+}-texaphyrin core conjugated to Dox were embedded. PEG and folate decorated surface of the liposome also provided tumor localization. Triggering ferroptosis, an iron-dependent programmed cell death mechanism, is an attractive approach. Yue *et al.* demonstrated an MRI contrast agent with face centered cubic FePt NPs that is conjugated to PTTA-Eu^{3+} complex and folate as a targeting moiety [30]. The PTTA-Eu^{3+} complex provided luminescent properties and it was possible to obtain MRI, CT as well as time gated-luminescence trimodal imaging modalities at the same time.

Radionuclide-based Imaging

Emission tomography (ET) is one of the favored imaging techniques in medicine that is depending on the detection of the radiation emitted by radioisotopes. In nuclear medicine, radiopharmaceuticals are used for positron emission tomography (PET) and single-photon emission computed tomography (SPECT) to obtain functional information to diagnose abnormalities of the tissues at cellular and molecular level [33].

PET imaging is based on positron emission and do not need an external stimulant, while SPECT is also a similar technique but it is based on detection of gamma rays by using gamma cameras and ring-type imaging systems [34]. Anatomical imaging is not possible with PET and SPECT. Therefore, the technique is combined with CT to obtain detailed information both from tissue and bones [35]. In "nano" image-based drug delivery systems, isotopes are conjugated on the surface of NPs. The main goal of using a NP conjugated with a radiolabel is the investigation of the therapeutic agent's distribution and targeting efficiency, stability in blood circulation, monitoring the response of the tumors and penetration in tumor tissue [36]. ^{18}F, ^{11}C, ^{15}O, ^{13}N, ^{64}Cu, ^{124}I, ^{68}Ga, ^{82}Rb, and ^{86}Y are the most common isotopes used in PET imaging. ^{123}I, ^{125}I, ^{99m}Tc, ^{111}In, ^{188}Re are the widely-used isotopes in SPECT imaging. These isotopes have longer half-life that allows longer time scanning compared to PET. Although, using positrons with short half-life decrease the imaging period, it increases the sensitivity incredibly in PET compared to SPECT. However, SPECT also has an advantage by the possibility of utilizing multiple isotopes, which make emissions at different energy levels contrary to positrons [34].

Gold NPs (AuNPs) are used as contrast agents and biosensors with their plasmonic properties. Both the surface characteristics of AuNPs that is allowing further surface modifications with stable thiol bonding, and the applications of radioactive labeling of AuNPs by neutron activation are special properties of AuNPs that widen their use in imaging-guided drug delivery and therapy [37]. A PEG-coated gold nanorod anti-cancer drug Dox-carrier conjugated with cyclo(Arg-Gly-Asp-D-Phe-Cys) peptides (cRGD) for tumor targeting and ^{64}Cu-chelators for PET imaging was reported. The drug release step was designed to have pH-dependent cleavable hydrazine bonds between nanocarrier and anti-cancer drug. Also in the study, the effect of cRGD conjugation specific to $\alpha v \beta 3$ was investigated and it was reported that targeting has no significant influence on tumor uptake in an *in vivo* study contrary to *in vitro* results due to the enhanced permeability and retention (EPR) effect.

The particles larger than 10 nm can enter into the tumor interstitials easily with the hyper-permeability property of tumor tissues. Also, molecules can be stable in tumors due to the lack of lymphatics. The gaps in tumors can be nearly a hundred nanometers, which is almost ten times higher than healthy tissues based on the interstitials between endothelial cells in tumors [38 - 40]. The EPR effect can give opportunity to the molecules with specific sizes to accumulate excessively in tumors, which can be an advantage in drug delivery by reducing the side effects of drugs on healthy cells.

Polymer-drug conjugations are generally used based on their long-term stability in blood circulation, low toxicity and allowing surface alterations for molecular targeting [41, 42]. N-(2-hydroxypropyl) methacrylamide (HPMA) is almost the most widely used polymer with its biocompatible properties [43 - 45]. Although the hydrophilic property of the HPMA limits its efficiency on lipophilic cell membranes, functionalization of the polymer backbone with a lipophilic lauryl methacrylate (LMA) can improve delivery [46, 47]. In a study of Allmeroth *et al.*, LMA modified HPMA was used as a drug carrier and conjugated with ^{18}F for PET imaging in two different tumor models; AT1 prostate carcinoma and Walker-256 mammary carcinoma [48]. The study demonstrates that the tumor model is the primary determinant with the polymer size and molecular weight for tumor accumulation. The results point out the requirement of designing personalized theranostic NPs for an efficient treatment.

Inorganic NPs such as silica and zeolite are used as drug carriers with their high loading capacity and their porous surface properties that allow efficient drug release [49]. PEG-coated mesoporous silica NPs, loaded with Dox were used as a tumor targeting PET imaging agent with ^{64}Cu labelling and TRC105 antibody conjugate targeted to CD105/endoglin, which is a vascular target for tumors, on 4T1 murine breast tumor in mice [50]. The efficiency of tumor vascular targeting depending on tumor cell type was demonstrated in the study. Highly stable ^{64}Cu labelling gave opportunity to monitor the distribution of nano platform and NP uptake with PET, non-invasively. The comparison of PET scans of TRC105-conjugated, untargeted and TRC105-blocked silica nano platform can be seen on Fig. (**2**). It is significantly seen that TRC105 conjugation increase the tumor uptake and tumor area becomes visible at 0.5 h. Also, renal clearance of NPs is one of the main challenges for clinical applications. Although there are contrary remarks about this for silica NPs, in a study by Chen *et al.*, they showed high accumulation in kidneys histologically [51]. It has to be also noted that, tumor vascular affinity of NPs is changing depending on tumor type and also most importantly from patient-to-patient. Indeed, development specific theranostic imaging nano designs within the scope of personalized medicine would cause successful treatment.

Liposomal NPs are used as very attractive drug conjugation systems and especially thermosensitive liposomes are used in temperature dependent drug release mechanisms [52]. ^{89}Zr is preferred with its strong gamma emission property and ^{89}Zr-conjugated liposomes are already manufactured by GE Fast Lab® and Eckert & Ziegler Modular Lab® for clinical use. Deferoxamine (DFO) loaded ^{89}Zr-liposomes used in a study with folic acid conjugated for targeted delivery as seen in the schematic illustration in Fig. (**3**) [53]. Unexpectedly, untargeted ^{89}Zr-liposomes are highly uploaded by KB tumors according to targeted liposomes, which again demonstrated that the EPR effect can be much more efficient than specific targeting. On the other hand, quantitative pharmacokinetics of liposomal drug carrier was determined with PET imaging in that study. The radioactive label is cleaned from kidney, liver and tumor but significant accumulation in bone was observed. It can be said that the main drawback of liposomal designs is their excess endothelial uptake, which cause catabolism and ion release (^{89}Zr) and bone uploading prevents the overall monitoring of liposomal drug carrier system circulation [53].

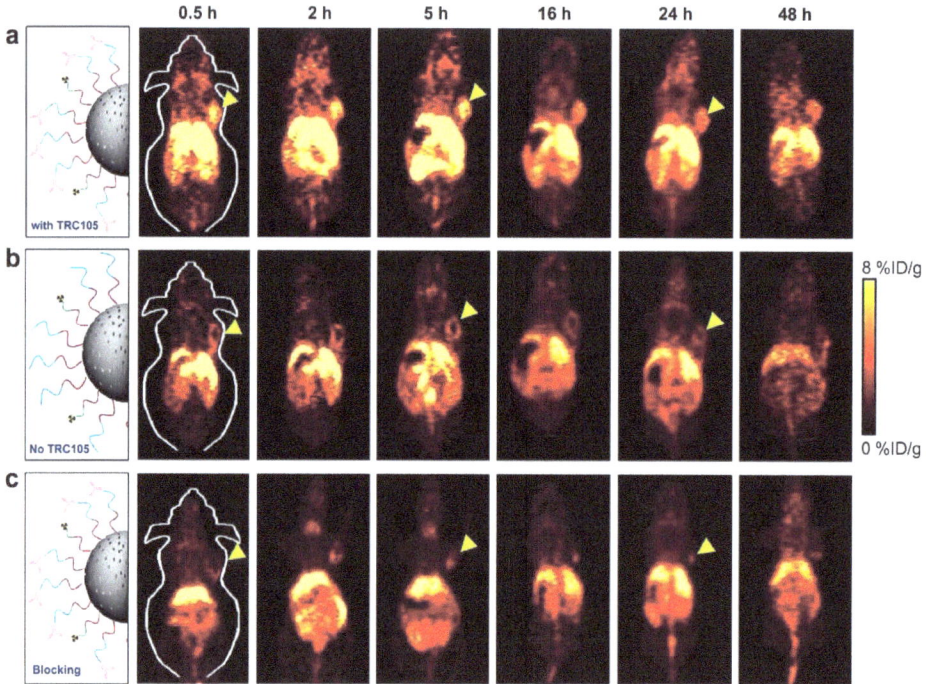

Fig. (2). Serial coronal PET images of 4T1 tumor-bearing mice at different time points postinjection of (a) ^{64}Cu-NOTA-mSiO$_2$-PEG-TRC105, (b) ^{64}Cu-NOTA-mSiO$_2$-PEG, or (c) ^{64}Cu-NOTA-mSiO$_2$-PEG-TRC105 with a blocking dose of TRC105. Tumors were indicated by yellow arrowheads. Reprinted with permission from (Chen *et al.*, 2013) [50]. Copyright 2013 American Chemical Society.

Radiopharmaceuticals are used for both their diagnostic and therapeutic properties. They are generally used with imaging techniques to allow monitoring the circulation and accumulation of the radiopharmaceutical in the body. In a study of Tsai *et al.*, micro SPECT/CT imaging technique was used to obtain detailed information about the drug targeting efficiency of a new PEGylated nanoliposome labelled with ^{188}Re according to conventional chemotherapeutic 5-fluorouracil (5-FU) in a C26 colonic peritoneal carcinomatosis mouse model [54]. ^{188}Re has advantages with its short half-life and long penetration depth and is a promising candidate in clinical use [55]. Also, it was demonstrated that intravenous injection is suitable for fast accumulation of radiopharmaceuticals to the target tissue [54].

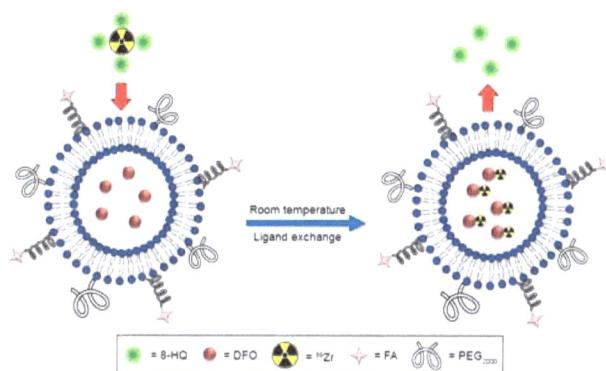

Fig. (3). [89]Zr labeling of an FA-decorated FA-DFO-liposome through a room-temperature ligand exchange reaction between the 89Zr(8-HQ)4 complex and the encapsulated DFO in the liposomal aqueous cavity. Abbreviations: FA, folic acid; DFO, deferoxamine; 8-HQ, 8-hydroxyquinoline; Abbreviations: FA, folic acid; DFO, deferoxamine; 8-HQ, 8-hydroxyquinoline; PEG 2000, (polyethylene glycol)-2000. Reprinted with permission from (Li *et al.*, 2017) [53]. Copyright 2013 Int J Nanomedicine. https://www.dovepress.com/ageneric- 89zr-labeling-method-to-quantify-the-*in-vivo*-pharmacokietic- peer-reviewed-article-IJN.

Angiogenesis is the formation of new blood vessels and has a primary role in tumor growth and avβ3 integrins are one of the contributing factors for this process. RGD peptides (Arg-Gly-Asp) can be used for selective targeting of these integrins and they were conjugated to AuNPs radiolabeled with ^{99m}Tc and used as a radiopharmaceutical in an *in vivo* study [56]. In this study, Morales-Avila *et al.* used micro SPECT/CT and showed tumor angiogenesis with high spatial resolution and in-depth analysis. It has to be noted that RGD conjugation and NP design increased tumor uptake significantly because this nano-system could not pass through whole cells easily due to their large size and accumulated in tumor significantly by targeting.

Drug retention time in tumor tissue is the primary determinant in cancer treatment. The drug molecules are often not stable in tumor tissue, drug resistance proteins send drugs back to the bloodstream [57, 58]. The main focus on the research studies is the enhancement of the drug retention time through both by intravenous and intratumor injections. In a recent study, iRGD porous silicon NPs were used for targeted delivery and loaded with sorafenib, hydrophobic antiangiogenic drug. The tumor uptake was followed by SPECT/CT imaging upon labelling the NPs with [111]In [59]. Sorafenib-loaded porous silicon NPs inhibited tumor growth significantly compared to free sorafenib. Although iRGD conjugation enhanced tumor accumulation and retention time as demonstrated in

SPECT/CT images, it still need improvements in delivering design. Currently, this is a very challenging topic in nanomedicine studies which needs to be solved.

Silver NPs (AgNPs) are one of the most studied materials with their optical properties and easy functionalization due to their active surface, which makes them an interested material in biomedical applications [60]. They are generally used with a polymeric shell on their outer surface and this shell improves permeability into the cells with the influence of EPR effect [61]. In a nano-based theranostic study, they used driving force of ^{125}I-labelled Dox-conjugated polyvinylpyrrolidone (PVP)-coated AgNPs on tumor therapy [62]. It was clearly indicated that this radiotheranostic delivery system achieved both tumor targeting and remaining in circulation system compared to both ^{125}I-labelled AgNPs and ^{125}I-labelled PVP-coated AgNPs.

In targeted drug delivery, the drug loading capacity, stability in blood circulation and drug release are indispensable for an efficient therapy. The hydrophobic interaction of drugs with NP through π-π stacking provide high drug loading capacity with large surface area of NPs as demonstrated in an *in vivo* colorectal cancer nano-therapy study [63]. cRGD modified polytyrosine NPs were used as a targeted drug carrier and Dox release was achieved by enzymatic degradation of the PEG and polystyrene diblock copolymer on the targeted cancer cells. The results proved that cRGD decoration increased the transferred drug amount from 41.3% to 72.9%, whereas it inhibited the tumor growth efficiently compared to untargeted design. The efficient accumulation of targeted nano Dox-carrier compared to un-targeted form was monitored with SPECT/CT through labelling with ^{125}I. It has to be also noted that such a theranostic design of Dox conjugation decreased the systematic toxicity as observed in using liposomal Dox.

X-Ray Computed Tomography

X-ray computed tomography (CT) is another widely used imaging technique in clinical diagnosis of severe diseases with its low cost and high spatial resolution compared to the other imaging techniques. The already used iodine-based contrast agents have disadvantages such as short half-life and side effects, which changed the scope of the recent research studies to find new alternatives [64, 65]. Gold, bismuth, tantalum, zirconium, silver and gadolinium-based NPs are the main NPs used in very recent studies with their CT imaging and drug delivering properties [66 - 74].

In the study of Hu *et al.*, Dox-loaded bismuth subcarbonate nanotubes were used as tumor targeting CT imaging and chemotherapeutic agent [66]. Bismuth-based nanotubes were used for their degradation property under acidic conditions, which not only allowed an efficient drug release but also provided excellent renal clearance. High drug loading capacity of the nano designs is very important for an efficient therapy using minimal amount of NPs. The researchers used hollow structured nanotubes with high-loading drug capacity. Also, the elongated structure of the nanotubes increased the tumor targeting efficiency. In a comprehensive study, PVP-coated porous bismuth nanospheres used for tumor imaging with CT and as a Dox-carrier for cancer therapy. Through the light absorption property of bismuth in the near infrared region (NIR), the possibility of applying PTT and radiotherapy besides chemotherapy was demonstrated. Also, it was shown that the NIR irradiation helped drug release in tumor area besides pH-dependent drug release [72].

AuNPs is an excellent X-ray contrast agent compared to iodine with its plasmonic property of rich electron environment, biocompatibility, non-toxicity and solubility [75 - 77]. The surface structure of AuNPs allowed further surface modifications for tumor targeting through thiol modifications without using any toxic bonding chemicals. Several cancer therapy studies demonstrated the potential of AuNPs as an imaging and drug delivery agent [67 - 69, 73]. In a study, AuNPs were prepared with using bovine serum albumin (BSA) and a stable and an efficient theranostic property of Dox and folic acid-conjugated design was demonstrated as seen in schematic illustration in Fig. (**4**) [67]. pH-sensitive chemotherapy in gastric cancer is achieved successfully in that study once again. Different from this study, Keshavarz and her colleagues used AuNPs as CT contrast agent but this time they used alginate for drug encapsulation [68]. It is known that the main goal in these designs is preventing the drug-healthy tissue interaction as much as possible. Therefore, they used hydrophilic and biocompatible alginate for drug encapsulation and followed the drug circulation with CT imaging. In a study of Lin *et al.* micellar formulation of AuNPs were used with 21-arm star like polymer β-cyclodextrin-{poly(ε-caprolactone)-po-y(2-aminoethyl methacrylate)-poly[poly(ethylene glycol) methyl ether methacrylate]}. The hydrophobic part of the micelle provided drug carrying and included a pH-sensitive part for drug release while, the hydrophilic part increased the blood circulation of the micellar design [69]. Using AuNPs in cluster form can be another way to target tumors with EPR effect and also the cluster form can be easily degraded and release the drug compared to particle form of the same size gold [73].

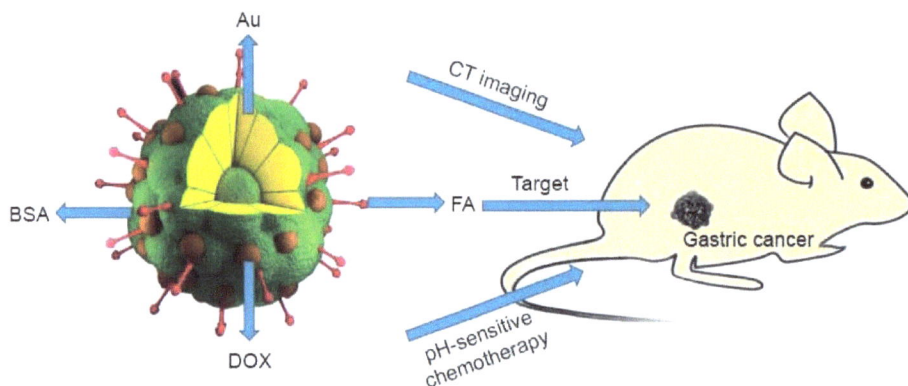

Fig. (4). Schematic diagram of an Au–BSA –DOX–FA nanocomposite model and multifunction in CT imaging and targeted therapy in FR-overexpressing gastric cancer xenografted mice. Abbreviations: BSA, bovine serum albumin; DOX, doxorubicin; FA, folic acid; CT, computed tomography; FR, folate receptor. Reprinted with permission from (Huang *et al.*, 2017) [67]. Copyright 2017 Int J Nanomedicine. https://www.dovepress.com/ph-sensitiv--aundashbsandashdoxndashf--nanocomposites-for-c-mbined-ct--peer-reviewed-article-IJN.

Tantalum is a relatively biocompatible transition metal, which is also widely used in biomedical applications [78]. It is used as a CT contrast agent and also tantalium sulfide form of the metal allows NIR absorption with its low band gap area [79]. Nanosheet form of tantalium sulfide was used in a recent study with its CT imaging and drug delivery properties [70]. Moreover, NIR irradiation enhanced the drug release from the nano platform efficiently. Most important outcome in this research study is the demonstration of the longer circulation time of tantalium compared to commercial CT contrast agent iobitridol used in the clinics.

Zirconium oxide NPs (ZrO_2 NPs), as a good alternative to iodine compounds, were used in a recent study [71]. They designed the ZrO_2 NPs in layer-by-layer formation and tested the synergistic effect of both thermotherapy with microwave ablation and chemotherapy by using Dox. In addition, acidic pH near tumor tissue increased the drug release significantly together with the effect of microwave.

Combination of imaging techniques by using multi-functional NP designs is possible and offers more information. In study published by Misra *et al.*, chitosan and Dox-conjugated bimetallic silver-gadolinium nanoarrays were prepared, which allowed employing CT and MRI techniques together [74]. These combined systems can provide opportunity to monitor drug delivery, drug release, and therapeutic effect both in anatomical and soft tissue examination.

CONCLUDING REMARKS

Multi-functional theranostic NPs are promising candidates in treatment of severe diseases as cancer with their advantageous properties such as high potential in targeted accumulation, drug delivery, and drug activation all of which can be monitored human body by the help of imaging modalities.

Although clinical trials with these particles seem possible in the near future, there are still issues to be cleared out. Safety and biocompatibility of NPs and challenges in synthesis procedures such as repeatability, scale-up and reaction yield of the complex designs are the handicaps that must be overcome before entering in clinical trials. In addition, coating process can decrease plasmonic or magnetic properties of NPs. Therefore, optimization of modification process should be performed definitely.

Currently, many improvements need to be done in the field which will then open the way up for the development of personalized medicine that will enable much more efficient therapy.

CONSENT FOR PUBLICATION

Not applicable.

CONFLICT OF INTEREST

The authors confirm that the contents of this chapter have no conflict of interest.

ACKNOWLEDGEMENTS

Declared none.

REFERENCES

[1]   Delli Castelli D, Dastrù W, Terreno E, *et al. In vivo* MRI multicontrast kinetic analysis of the uptake and intracellular trafficking of paramagnetically labeled liposomes. J Control Release 2010; 144(3): 271-9.
[http://dx.doi.org/10.1016/j.jconrel.2010.03.005] [PMID: 20230865]

[2]   Kato Y, Artemov D. Monitoring of release of cargo from nanocarriers by MRI/MR spectroscopy (MRS): significance of T2/T2* effect of iron particles. Magn Reson Med 2009; 61(5): 1059-65.
[http://dx.doi.org/10.1002/mrm.21939] [PMID: 19253373]

[3]   Langereis S, Keupp J, van Velthoven JL, *et al.* A temperature-sensitive liposomal 1H CEST and 19F contrast agent for MR image-guided drug delivery. J Am Chem Soc 2009; 131(4): 1380-1.
[http://dx.doi.org/10.1021/ja8087532] [PMID: 19173663]

[4]   Chen T, Shukoor MI, Wang R, *et al.* Smart multifunctional nanostructure for targeted cancer chemotherapy and magnetic resonance imaging. ACS Nano 2011; 5(10): 7866-73.
[http://dx.doi.org/10.1021/nn202073m] [PMID: 21888350]

[5] Lee GY, Qian WP, Wang L, *et al.* Theranostic nanoparticles with controlled release of gemcitabine for targeted therapy and MRI of pancreatic cancer. ACS Nano 2013; 7(3): 2078-89.
[http://dx.doi.org/10.1021/nn3043463] [PMID: 23402593]

[6] Willerding L, Limmer S, Hossann M, *et al.* Method of hyperthermia and tumor size influence effectiveness of doxorubicin release from thermosensitive liposomes in experimental tumors. J Control Release 2016; 222: 47-55.
[http://dx.doi.org/10.1016/j.jconrel.2015.12.004] [PMID: 26658073]

[7] Guo Y, Zhang Y, Ma J, *et al.* Light/magnetic hyperthermia triggered drug released from multi-functional thermo-sensitive magnetoliposomes for precise cancer synergetic theranostics. J Control Release 2018; 272: 145-58.
[http://dx.doi.org/10.1016/j.jconrel.2017.04.028] [PMID: 28442407]

[8] Rizzitelli S, Giustetto P, Boffa C, *et al. In vivo* MRI visualization of release from liposomes triggered by local application of pulsed low-intensity non-focused ultrasound. Nanomedicine (Lond) 2014; 10(5): 901-4.
[http://dx.doi.org/10.1016/j.nano.2014.03.012] [PMID: 24657833]

[9] Lux F, Tran VL, Thomas E, *et al.* AGuIX((R)) from bench to bedside-Transfer of an ultrasmall theranostic gadolinium-based nanoparticle to clinical medicine. Br J Radiol 2019; 92(1093): 20180365.
[http://dx.doi.org/10.1259/bjr.20180365] [PMID: 30226413]

[10] Yang JC, Shang Y, Li YH, Cui Y, Yin XB. An "all-in-one" antitumor and anti-recurrence/metastasis nanomedicine with multi-drug co-loading and burst drug release for multi-modality therapy. Chem Sci (Camb) 2018; 9(36): 7210-7.
[http://dx.doi.org/10.1039/C8SC02305K] [PMID: 30288240]

[11] Zhang H, Liu K, Li S, *et al.* Self-assembled minimalist multifunctional theranostic nanoplatform for magnetic resonance imaging-guided tumor photodynamic therapy. ACS Nano 2018; 12(8): 8266-76.
[http://dx.doi.org/10.1021/acsnano.8b03529] [PMID: 30091901]

[12] Li NN, Cheng JJ, Zhang Y, Wang J, Huang G, Zhu J, *et al.* A chemophotothermal and targeting multifunctional nanoprobe with a tumor-diagnosing ability. Nano Res 2018; 11: 4333-47.
[http://dx.doi.org/10.1007/s12274-018-2021-0]

[13] Cheng L, Yang K, Li Y, *et al.* Facile preparation of multifunctional upconversion nanoprobes for multimodal imaging and dual-targeted photothermal therapy. Angew Chem Int Ed Engl 2011; 50(32): 7385-90.
[http://dx.doi.org/10.1002/anie.201101447] [PMID: 21714049]

[14] Kenny GD, Kamaly N, Kalber TL, *et al.* Novel multifunctional nanoparticle mediates siRNA tumour delivery, visualisation and therapeutic tumour reduction *in vivo.* J Control Release 2011; 149(2): 111-6.
[http://dx.doi.org/10.1016/j.jconrel.2010.09.020] [PMID: 20888381]

[15] Wu B, Wan B, Lu ST, *et al.* Near-infrared light-triggered theranostics for tumor-specific enhanced multimodal imaging and photothermal therapy. Int J Nanomed 2017; 12: 4467-78.
[http://dx.doi.org/10.2147/IJN.S137835] [PMID: 28670120]

[16] Yang JC, Chen Y, Li YH, Yin XB. Magnetic resonance imaging-guided multi-drug chemotherapy and photothermal synergistic therapy with pH and NIR-stimulation release. ACS Appl Mater Interfaces 2017; 9(27): 22278-88.
[http://dx.doi.org/10.1021/acsami.7b06105] [PMID: 28616966]

[17] Kwon YS, Jang SJ, Yoon YI, *et al.* Magnetic liposomal particles for magnetic imaging, sensing, and the pH-sensitive delivery of therapeutics. Part Part Syst Charact 2016; 33: 242-7.
[http://dx.doi.org/10.1002/ppsc.201600041]

[18] Semkina AS, Abakumov MA, Skorikov AS, *et al.* Multimodal doxorubicin loaded magnetic

nanoparticles for VEGF targeted theranostics of breast cancer. Nanomedicine (Lond) 2018; 14(5): 1733-42.
[http://dx.doi.org/10.1016/j.nano.2018.04.019] [PMID: 29730399]

[19]　Yue L, Wang J, Dai Z, *et al.* pH-responsive, self-sacrificial nanotheranostic agent for potential *in vivo* and *in vitro* dual modal MRI/CT imaging, real-time, and *in situ* monitoring of cancer therapy. Bioconjug Chem 2017; 28(2): 400-9.
[http://dx.doi.org/10.1021/acs.bioconjchem.6b00562] [PMID: 28042941]

[20]　de Smet M, Heijman E, Langereis S, Hijnen NM, Grüll H. Magnetic resonance imaging of high intensity focused ultrasound mediated drug delivery from temperature-sensitive liposomes: an *in vivo* proof-of-concept study. J Control Release 2011; 150(1): 102-10.
[http://dx.doi.org/10.1016/j.jconrel.2010.10.036] [PMID: 21059375]

[21]　Lee MH, Kim EJ, Lee H, *et al.* Liposomal texaphyrin theranostics for metastatic liver cancer. J Am Chem Soc 2016; 138(50): 16380-7.
[http://dx.doi.org/10.1021/jacs.6b09713] [PMID: 27998081]

[22]　Saesoo S, Sathornsumetee S, Anekwiang P, *et al.* Characterization of liposome-containing SPIONs conjugated with anti-CD20 developed as a novel theranostic agent for central nervous system lymphoma. Colloids Surf B Biointerfaces 2018; 161: 497-507.
[http://dx.doi.org/10.1016/j.colsurfb.2017.11.003] [PMID: 29128836]

[23]　Zheng XC, Ren W, Zhang S, *et al.* The theranostic efficiency of tumor-specific, pH-responsive, peptide-modified, liposome-containing paclitaxel and superparamagnetic iron oxide nanoparticles. Int J Nanomed 2018; 13: 1495-504.
[http://dx.doi.org/10.2147/IJN.S157082] [PMID: 29559778]

[24]　Kostarelos K, Miller AD. Synthetic, self-assembly ABCD nanoparticles; a structural paradigm for viable synthetic non-viral vectors. Chem Soc Rev 2005; 34(11): 970-94.
[http://dx.doi.org/10.1039/b307062j] [PMID: 16239997]

[25]　Liu G, Ma J, Li Y, *et al.* Core-interlayer-shell Fe_3O_4@mSiO_2@lipid-PEG-methotrexate nanoparticle for multimodal imaging and multistage targeted chemo-photodynamic therapy. Int J Pharm 2017; 521(1-2): 19-32.
[http://dx.doi.org/10.1016/j.ijpharm.2017.01.068] [PMID: 28163230]

[26]　Perlman O, Weitz IS, Sivan SS, *et al.* Copper oxide loaded PLGA nanospheres: towards a multifunctional nanoscale platform for ultrasound-based imaging and therapy. Nanotechnology 2018; 29(18): 185102.
[http://dx.doi.org/10.1088/1361-6528/aab00c] [PMID: 29451124]

[27]　Tang H, Guo Y, Peng L, *et al. In vivo* targeted, responsive, and synergistic cancer nanotheranostics by magnetic resonance imaging-guided synergistic high-intensity focused ultrasound ablation and chemotherapy. ACS Appl Mater Interfaces 2018; 10(18): 15428-41.
[http://dx.doi.org/10.1021/acsami.8b01967] [PMID: 29652130]

[28]　Mrówczyński R. Polydopamine-Based Multifunctional (Nano)materials for Cancer Therapy. ACS Appl Mater Interfaces 2018; 10(9): 7541-61.
[http://dx.doi.org/10.1021/acsami.7b08392] [PMID: 28786657]

[29]　Wang D, Zhou J, Chen R, *et al.* Controllable synthesis of dual-MOFs nanostructures for pH-responsive artemisinin delivery, magnetic resonance and optical dual-model imaging-guided chemo/photothermal combinational cancer therapy. Biomaterials 2016; 100: 27-40.
[http://dx.doi.org/10.1016/j.biomaterials.2016.05.027] [PMID: 27240160]

[30]　Yue L, Dai Z, Chen X, *et al.* Development of a novel FePt-based multifunctional ferroptosis agent for high-efficiency anticancer therapy. Nanoscale 2018; 10(37): 17858-64.
[http://dx.doi.org/10.1039/C8NR05150J] [PMID: 30221289]

[31]　Li B, Tang J, Chen W, *et al.* Novel theranostic nanoplatform for complete mice tumor elimination *via* MR imaging-guided acid-enhanced photothermo-/chemo-therapy. Biomaterials 2018; 177: 40-51.

[http://dx.doi.org/10.1016/j.biomaterials.2018.05.055] [PMID: 29883915]

[32]   Zhang Q, Shan W, Ai C, *et al.* Construction of Multifunctional Fe$_3$O$_4$-MTX@HBc Nanoparticles for MR Imaging and Photothermal Therapy/Chemotherapy. Nanotheranostics 2018; 2(1): 87-95.
[http://dx.doi.org/10.7150/ntno.21942] [PMID: 29291165]

[33]   Spencer SS, Theodore WH, Berkovic SF. Clinical applications: MRI, SPECT, and PET. Magn Reson Imaging 1995; 13(8): 1119-24.
[http://dx.doi.org/10.1016/0730-725X(95)02021-K] [PMID: 8750325]

[34]   Hahn MA, Singh AK, Sharma P, Brown SC, Moudgil BM. Nanoparticles as contrast agents for *in vivo* bioimaging: current status and future perspectives. Anal Bioanal Chem 2011; 399(1): 3-27.
[http://dx.doi.org/10.1007/s00216-010-4207-5] [PMID: 20924568]

[35]   Massoud TF, Gambhir SS. Molecular imaging in living subjects: seeing fundamental biological processes in a new light. Genes Dev 2003; 17(5): 545-80.
[http://dx.doi.org/10.1101/gad.1047403] [PMID: 12629038]

[36]   Benezra M, Penate-Medina O, Zanzonico PB, *et al.* Multimodal silica nanoparticles are effective cancer-targeted probes in a model of human melanoma. J Clin Invest 2011; 121(7): 2768-80.
[http://dx.doi.org/10.1172/JCI45600] [PMID: 21670497]

[37]   Kong FY, Zhang JW, Li RF, Wang ZX, Wang WJ, Wang W. Unique Roles of Gold Nanoparticles in Drug Delivery, Targeting and Imaging Applications. Molecules 2017; 22(9): 22.
[PMID: 28858253]

[38]   Hobbs SK, Monsky WL, Yuan F, *et al.* Regulation of transport pathways in tumor vessels: role of tumor type and microenvironment. Proc Natl Acad Sci USA 1998; 95(8): 4607-12.
[http://dx.doi.org/10.1073/pnas.95.8.4607] [PMID: 9539785]

[39]   Jain RK, Stylianopoulos T. Delivering nanomedicine to solid tumors. Nat Rev Clin Oncol 2010; 7(11): 653-64.
[http://dx.doi.org/10.1038/nrclinonc.2010.139] [PMID: 20838415]

[40]   Sarin H. Physiologic upper limits of pore size of different blood capillary types and another perspective on the dual pore theory of microvascular permeability. J Angiogenes Res 2010; 2: 14.
[http://dx.doi.org/10.1186/2040-2384-2-14] [PMID: 20701757]

[41]   Lammers T. Improving the efficacy of combined modality anticancer therapy using HPMA copolymer-based nanomedicine formulations. Adv Drug Deliv Rev 2010; 62(2): 203-30.
[http://dx.doi.org/10.1016/j.addr.2009.11.028] [PMID: 19951732]

[42]   Pike DB, Ghandehari H. HPMA copolymer-cyclic RGD conjugates for tumor targeting. Adv Drug Deliv Rev 2010; 62(2): 167-83.
[http://dx.doi.org/10.1016/j.addr.2009.11.027] [PMID: 19951733]

[43]   Janib SM, Moses AS, MacKay JA. Imaging and drug delivery using theranostic nanoparticles. Adv Drug Deliv Rev 2010; 62(11): 1052-63.
[http://dx.doi.org/10.1016/j.addr.2010.08.004] [PMID: 20709124]

[44]   Kopecek J, Kopecková P. HPMA copolymers: origins, early developments, present, and future. Adv Drug Deliv Rev 2010; 62(2): 122-49.
[http://dx.doi.org/10.1016/j.addr.2009.10.004] [PMID: 19919846]

[45]   Lammers T, Ulbrich K. HPMA copolymers: 30 years of advances. Adv Drug Deliv Rev 2010; 62(2): 119-21.
[http://dx.doi.org/10.1016/j.addr.2009.12.004] [PMID: 20005273]

[46]   Hemmelmann M, Knoth C, Schmitt U, *et al.* HPMA based amphiphilic copolymers mediate central nervous effects of domperidone. Macromol Rapid Commun 2011; 32(9-10): 712-7.
[http://dx.doi.org/10.1002/marc.201000810] [PMID: 21469240]

[47]   Hemmelmann M, Metz VV, Koynov K, Blank K, Postina R, Zentel R. Amphiphilic HPMA-LMA

copolymers increase the transport of Rhodamine 123 across a BBB model without harming its barrier integrity. J Control Release 2012; 163(2): 170-7.
[http://dx.doi.org/10.1016/j.jconrel.2012.08.034] [PMID: 22981565]

[48] Allmeroth M, Moderegger D, Gündel D, *et al.* HPMA-LMA copolymer drug carriers in oncology: an *in vivo* PET study to assess the tumor line-specific polymer uptake and body distribution. Biomacromolecules 2013; 14(9): 3091-101.
[http://dx.doi.org/10.1021/bm400709z] [PMID: 23962188]

[49] Tarn D, Ashley CE, Xue M, Carnes EC, Zink JI, Brinker CJ. Mesoporous silica nanoparticle nanocarriers: biofunctionality and biocompatibility. Acc Chem Res 2013; 46(3): 792-801.
[http://dx.doi.org/10.1021/ar3000986] [PMID: 23387478]

[50] Chen F, Hong H, Zhang Y, *et al. In vivo* tumor targeting and image-guided drug delivery with antibody-conjugated, radiolabeled mesoporous silica nanoparticles. ACS Nano 2013; 7(10): 9027-39.
[http://dx.doi.org/10.1021/nn403617j] [PMID: 24083623]

[51] Chen F, Nayak TR, Goel S, *et al. In vivo* tumor vasculature targeted PET/NIRF imaging with TRC105(Fab)-conjugated, dual-labeled mesoporous silica nanoparticles. Mol Pharm 2014; 11(11): 4007-14.
[http://dx.doi.org/10.1021/mp500306k] [PMID: 24937108]

[52] Noble GT, Stefanick JF, Ashley JD, Kiziltepe T, Bilgicer B. Ligand-targeted liposome design: challenges and fundamental considerations. Trends Biotechnol 2014; 32(1): 32-45.
[http://dx.doi.org/10.1016/j.tibtech.2013.09.007] [PMID: 24210498]

[53] Li N, Yu Z, Pham TT, Blower PJ, Yan R. A generic ^{89}Zr labeling method to quantify the *in vivo* pharmacokinetics of liposomal nanoparticles with positron emission tomography. Int J Nanomed 2017; 12: 3281-94.
[http://dx.doi.org/10.2147/IJN.S134379] [PMID: 28458546]

[54] Tsai CC, Chang CH, Chen LC, *et al.* Biodistribution and pharmacokinetics of 188Re-liposomes and their comparative therapeutic efficacy with 5-fluorouracil in C26 colonic peritoneal carcinomatosis mice. Int J Nanomed 2011; 6: 2607-19.
[PMID: 22114492]

[55] Ting G, Chang CH, Wang HE. Cancer nanotargeted radiopharmaceuticals for tumor imaging and therapy. Anticancer Res 2009; 29(10): 4107-18.
[PMID: 19846958]

[56] Morales-Avila E, Ferro-Flores G, Ocampo-García BE, *et al.* Multimeric system of 99mTc-labeled gold nanoparticles conjugated to c[RGDfK(C)] for molecular imaging of tumor α(v)β(3) expression. Bioconjug Chem 2011; 22(5): 913-22.
[http://dx.doi.org/10.1021/bc100551s] [PMID: 21513349]

[57] Han HD, Byeon Y, Jeon HN, Shin BC. Enhanced localization of anticancer drug in tumor tissue using polyethylenimine-conjugated cationic liposomes. Nanoscale Res Lett 2014; 9(1): 209.
[http://dx.doi.org/10.1186/1556-276X-9-209] [PMID: 24855464]

[58] Nichols JW, Bae YH. EPR: Evidence and fallacy. J Control Release 2014; 190: 451-64.
[http://dx.doi.org/10.1016/j.jconrel.2014.03.057] [PMID: 24794900]

[59] Wang CF, Sarparanta MP, Mäkilä EM, *et al.* Multifunctional porous silicon nanoparticles for cancer theranostics. Biomaterials 2015; 48: 108-18.
[http://dx.doi.org/10.1016/j.biomaterials.2015.01.008] [PMID: 25701036]

[60] Burduşel AC, Gherasim O, Grumezescu AM, Mogoantă L, Ficai A, Andronescu E. Biomedical applications of silver nanoparticles: An up-to-date overview. Nanomaterials (Basel) 2018; 8(9): 8.
[http://dx.doi.org/10.3390/nano8090681] [PMID: 30200373]

[61] Soares DC, Ferreira TH, Ferreira CdeA, Cardoso VN, de Sousa EM. Boron nitride nanotubes radiolabeled with ^{99}mTc: preparation, physicochemical characterization, biodistribution study, and

scintigraphic imaging in Swiss mice. Int J Pharm 2012; 423(2): 489-95.
[http://dx.doi.org/10.1016/j.ijpharm.2011.12.002] [PMID: 22178127]

[62]   Farrag NS, El-Sabagh HA, Al-Mahallawi AM, Amin AM, AbdEl-Bary A, Mamdouh W. Comparative study on radiolabeling and biodistribution of core-shell silver/polymeric nanoparticles-based theranostics for tumor targeting. Int J Pharm 2017; 529(1-2): 123-33.
[http://dx.doi.org/10.1016/j.ijpharm.2017.06.044] [PMID: 28624660]

[63]   Gu X, Wei Y, Fan Q, *et al.* cRGD-decorated biodegradable polytyrosine nanoparticles for robust encapsulation and targeted delivery of doxorubicin to colorectal cancer *in vivo.* J Control Release 2019; 301: 110-8.
[http://dx.doi.org/10.1016/j.jconrel.2019.03.005] [PMID: 30898610]

[64]   Haller C, Hizoh I. The cytotoxicity of iodinated radiocontrast agents on renal cells *in vitro.* Invest Radiol 2004; 39(3): 149-54.
[http://dx.doi.org/10.1097/01.rli.0000113776.87762.49] [PMID: 15076007]

[65]   Hyafil F, Cornily JC, Feig JE, *et al.* Noninvasive detection of macrophages using a nanoparticulate contrast agent for computed tomography. Nat Med 2007; 13(5): 636-41.
[http://dx.doi.org/10.1038/nm1571] [PMID: 17417649]

[66]   Hu X, Sun J, Li F, *et al.* Renal-clearable hollow bismuth subcarbonate nanotubes for tumor targeted computed tomography imaging and chemoradiotherapy. Nano Lett 2018; 18(2): 1196-204.
[http://dx.doi.org/10.1021/acs.nanolett.7b04741] [PMID: 29297694]

[67]   Huang H, Yang DP, Liu M, *et al.* pH-sensitive Au-BSA-DOX-FA nanocomposites for combined CT imaging and targeted drug delivery. Int J Nanomed 2017; 12: 2829-43.
[http://dx.doi.org/10.2147/IJN.S128270] [PMID: 28435261]

[68]   Keshavarz M, Moloudi K, Paydar R, *et al.* Alginate hydrogel co-loaded with cisplatin and gold nanoparticles for computed tomography image-guided chemotherapy. J Biomater Appl 2018; 33(2): 161-9.
[http://dx.doi.org/10.1177/0885328218782355] [PMID: 29933708]

[69]   Lin W, Zhang X, Qian L, Yao N, Pan Y, Zhang L. Doxorubicin-Loaded unimolecular micelle-stabilized gold nanoparticles as a theranostic nanoplatform for tumor-targeted chemotherapy and computed tomography imaging. Biomacromolecules 2017; 18(12): 3869-80.
[http://dx.doi.org/10.1021/acs.biomac.7b00810] [PMID: 29032674]

[70]   Liu Y, Ji X, Liu J, Tong WWL, Askhatova D, Shi J. Tantalum sulfide nanosheets as a theranostic nanoplatform for computed tomography imaging-guided combinatorial chemo-photothermal therapy. Adv Funct Mater 2017; 27(39): 27.
[http://dx.doi.org/10.1002/adfm.201703261] [PMID: 29290753]

[71]   Long D, Niu M, Tan L, *et al.* Ball-in-ball ZrO_2 nanostructure for simultaneous CT imaging and highly efficient synergic microwave ablation and tri-stimuli-responsive chemotherapy of tumors. Nanoscale 2017; 9(25): 8834-47.
[http://dx.doi.org/10.1039/C7NR02511D] [PMID: 28632268]

[72]   Ma G, Liu X, Deng G, Yuan H, Wang Q, Lu J. A novel theranostic agent based on porous bismuth nanosphere for CT imaging-guided combined chemo-photothermal therapy and radiotherapy. J Mater Chem B Mater Biol Med 2018; 6(42): 6788-95.
[http://dx.doi.org/10.1039/C8TB02189A] [PMID: 32254695]

[73]   Mao W, Kim HS, Son YJ, Kim SR, Yoo HS. Doxorubicin encapsulated clicked gold nanoparticle clusters exhibiting tumor-specific disassembly for enhanced tumor localization and computerized tomographic imaging. J Control Release 2018; 269: 52-62.
[http://dx.doi.org/10.1016/j.jconrel.2017.11.003] [PMID: 29113793]

[74]   Mishra SK, Kannan S. Doxorubicin-conjugated bimetallic silver-gadolinium nanoalloy for multimodal MRI-CT-optical imaging and pH-responsive drug release. ACS Biomater Sci Eng 2017; 3: 3607-19.
[http://dx.doi.org/10.1021/acsbiomaterials.7b00498]

[75]   Chen CT, Chen WJ, Liu CZ, Chang LY, Chen YC. Glutathione-bound gold nanoclusters for selective-binding and detection of glutathione S-transferase-fusion proteins from cell lysates. Chem Commun (Camb) 2009; (48): 7515-7.
[http://dx.doi.org/10.1039/b916919a] [PMID: 20024264]

[76]   Song L, Guo Y, Roebuck D, *et al.* Terminal PEGylated DNA-gold nanoparticle conjugates offering high resistance to nuclease degradation and efficient intracellular deliveryof DNA binding agents. ACS Appl Mater Interfaces 2015; 7(33): 18707-16.
[http://dx.doi.org/10.1021/acsami.5b05228] [PMID: 26237203]

[77]   Sperling RA, Rivera Gil P, Zhang F, Zanella M, Parak WJ. Biological applications of gold nanoparticles. Chem Soc Rev 2008; 37(9): 1896-908.
[http://dx.doi.org/10.1039/b712170a] [PMID: 18762838]

[78]   Black J. Biological performance of tantalum. Clin Mater 1994; 16(3): 167-73.
[http://dx.doi.org/10.1016/0267-6605(94)90113-9] [PMID: 10172264]

[79]   Nguyen TP, Choi S, Jeon JM, Kwon KC, Jang HW, Kim SY. Transition metal disulfide nanosheets synthesized by facile sonication method for the hydrogen evolution reaction. J Phys Chem C 2016; 120: 3929-35.
[http://dx.doi.org/10.1021/acs.jpcc.5b12164]

CHAPTER 7

Practical Clinical Applications: Chemotherapy and Nuclear Medicine

Turkan Ikizceli[1,*] and **S. Karacavus**[2]

[1] *Department of Radiology, University of Health Sciences Turkey, Haseki Training and Research Hospital, Istanbul, Turkey*

[2] *Department of Nuclear Medicine, University of Health Sciences Turkey, Kayseri City Training and Research Hospital, Kayseri, Turkey*

Abstract: An optimized and particular cancer therapy must deliver the right type of treatment to the right targeted tissue to achieve control of the disease efficiently with minimal local and systemic toxicity and side effects. Advances in nanotechnology have introduced some approaches that offer new alternatives to diagnose and treat after being used in medicine. When the hydrophilic molecules are attached as carrier particles, they may remain in circulation for longer, which leads to the target organ. These new advances in recent years in nanotheranostics have expanded this concept and allowed characterization of individual tumors, prediction of nanoparticle–tumor interactions, and creation of tailor-designed new nanomedicines for individualized treatment in medicine. Advances in imaging technologies used in diseases, in general, have resulted in additional consortium guidelines for standardizing diagnostic imaging in clinical oncology. Diagnostic imaging using Ultrasonography (US), Computed Tomography (CT), Magnetic Resonance Imaging (MRI), and Positron Emission Tomography (PET) have been the most important tools. Nuclear Imaging allows a proper diagnosis, much earlier treatment, and better follow up opening a new door by non-invasive *in vitro/ex vivo* assessments in the oncology field and for personalized medicine. A nanotheranostic probe for nuclear medicine gives combined diagnostic and therapeutic capabilities by radiolabeling the different emitters (α, β^+, β^-, γ) used for imaging and/or therapy. The radiolabeled nanoparticles consist of the labeling of radionuclides onto the nanomaterials that cause deeper penetration increasing internal radiotherapy in cancer cells and inducing cell death. An ideal radionuclide nanotheranostic probe has properties such as long shelf life, easily accessible radionuclides, convenient half-life, easy and high marking efficiency, *in vivo* stability, lack of immunological reaction, rapidly clearance from circulation and directed to the target, high image quality, retention of radionuclide in the liposome and its metabolites should be non-toxic. The emergence and its further development of the nanotheranostic

---

* **Corresponding author Turkan Ikizceli:** Department of Radiology, University of Health Sciences Turkey, Haseki Training and Research Hospital, Istanbul, Turkey; E-mail: turkan.ikizceli@sbu.edu.tr

concept illustrate the need for a multidisciplinary approach with the common objective of improving the management of clinical oncology trials. The simultaneous yield of imaging in radiologic and nuclear medicine applications and therapeutic agents offer the possibility of diagnosis and treatment feedbacks on the treatment effectiveness in real-time.

Keywords: Cancer diagnosis, Cancer therapy, Chemotherapy, Computed tomography, Imaging modalities, Magnetic resonance imaging, Nanotheranostics, Nuclear medicine.

INTRODUCTION

Advances in nanotechnology have introduced some approaches that offer new alternatives in drug production, diagnosis, and treatment after being used in medicine [1]. The most crucial advantage of nanoparticles is that their particle size is very tiny. Due to their small size, the ability to easily pass through the vessels and circulation forms the basis of their usability in treatment. When the hydrophilic molecules are attached as carrier particles, they may remain longer in circulation. More than one active unit can be loaded on a carrier, and can be directed to the target organ [2]. This helps in the drug-release monitoring, imaging-guided local treatment, and post-treatment response monitoring and follow-up. Also, the progress of nanotheranostics has allowed the characterization of individual tumors, estimation between nanoparticles and intra-tumor interactions, and the formation of tailor-designed nanomedicines for individualized treatment. An optimized cancer therapy must deliver the right treatment design to the accurate target to have localized control of the disease with minimal systemic toxicity and side effects [3]. But in reality, there is significant variation among tumors and individual patients. It will require careful coordination of diagnosis and treatment, real identification of the patient and tumor subgroups, and medications. Developments in nanotechnology in medicine offer a promising opportunity for this new field and create a modern workplace. At the same time, treatment can be monitored non-invasively and in real-time. A traditional nanotheranostic agent is made by combining both diagnostic and therapeutic components [3].

Applications of Nanotheranostics in Cancer Chemotherapy

The combination of imaging and treatment using nanotechnology has become one of the forefront topics of research nowadays. In the last decade, plenty of nanoparticles have been developed for their potential applications as diagnostic and therapeutic agents. The use of nanotechnology in medicine, known as nanomedicine, has increased the interest, as a variable strategy for choosing the right drug delivery and diagnostic purposes. Nanotheranostics gives hope because it integrates the simultaneous and non-invasive diagnosis and treatment of diseases with the exciting possibility to monitor drug release and distribution in real-time, thus giving notice and confirming the impact of the procedure. These features of nanotheranostics are very engaging for optimizing therapy results in oncological clinical trials. The next step of the trial is using them for an accurate, personalized medicine that will adapt the optimized therapy to cancer patients [4].

Clinical application of nanotheranostics makes it possible to detect and treat cancer earlier, estimate, monitor, and screen patient responses to treatment [5].

An ideal nanotheranostic agent should have the following features: a) Ability to detect tumor location, b) High signal-to-noise ratio (SNR), c) High specificity for early detection, d) Non-toxic or at least minimal systemic toxicity at the concentration necessary for the diagnostic signal. These features make it possible (1) for early detection, (2) proper drug selection, (3) discovery of biomarkers, (4) staging of the disease, (5) monitoring drug release in real-time, and (6) determination of therapeutic outcomes during therapy and post-therapy [6].

The mechanism of traditional chemotherapy seeks to exploit the differences between cancer and healthy cells. Unfortunately, chemotherapeutic drugs still have high systemic toxicity and considerable morbidity in modern medicine. Due to this systemic toxicity, tumors rapidly develop resistance and limit the dosage of these drugs. Nanotherapeutics achieve a synergistic effect by blocking multiple receptors within cancer, reducing systemic toxicity by minimizing the dose of the medicine in the circulation. Furthermore, by combining these drugs with the target molecule, they specifically help to bind the targeted chemotherapeutic agent to cancer cells and increase the therapeutic index [7]. Although the effectiveness of nanotheranostics has been proved, many are still far from clinical practices. Treatment of cancer requires an accurate diagnosis and correct staging using a specific imaging method before planning the therapy.

Imaging plays the primary role in cancer diagnosing, staging, and monitoring in clinical trials. In recent years, a considerable number of new imaging technologies and targeted tracers have been developed for cancer imaging but are not yet in clinical use due to a lack of sufficient standards [8]. Also, personalized medicine is gaining immense importance. A particular type of treatment for a specific disease may be beneficial for one individual, but not for the other patients. The different responses of patients to the same procedure mostly depend on their genetic differences. Because of this variation, it is difficult to make an accurate prediction of many medical conditions [9, 10]. With the increase in personalized therapeutic approach, diagnostic methods and imaging modalities are of great help in providing reliable and early clinical phase assessments. Thus, an ideal nanotheranostics for theranostic purpose should provide safe, accurate diagnosis and imaging, individualized therapy, and evaluation of real-time therapeutic effects. Therefore, it is still a very challenging field and requires the development of new strategies and methods [11]. These include patient screening, diagnosis, treatment, and follow-up of cancer that can all be done with "image-guidance." The use of nanotheranostics makes it possible to screen, diagnose, and monitor biodistribution and target tissue accumulation. Among the imaging modalities, Magnetic resonance imaging (MRI) and Computed Tomography (CT) are the two main imaging techniques currently used for diagnostic purposes in oncologic disease evaluation [12, 13].

MRI, as the most potent non-invasive imaging technique in clinical medicine, has been widely used in diagnosis because of its high spatial resolution for soft tissues, noninvasiveness, and excellent tissue penetration. The tissue signal of the image in MRI originates from water protons, and this intrinsic contrast is known as "proton density contrast." Each tissue has its relaxation times. Different T1 (longitudinal) and T2 (transverse) proton relaxation times in these tissues produce endogenous contrast [14]. However, MRI has reduced sensitivity and might prevent accurate tumor diagnosis. It is not efficient to differentiate between healthy soft tissues and/or tumors [15].

For this reason, an MRI examination in cancer treatment requires an exogenous contrast agent containing gadolinium. Contrast agents reduce relaxation time for both the T1 and T2 sequences, leading to a bright (positive) or dark (negative) contrast enhancement. Different contrast agents are used for T1 and T2 sequences, while paramagnetic metal ions such as Gd^{3+}, manganese (Mn^{2+} and Mn^{3+}) are used as T1 contrast agents, iron oxide NPs are the most used as T2 contrast agents. Also, contrast agents are used to increase the contrast between tissues and reduce SNR, thereby increasing detection sensitivity. Although it is valuable to use contrast agents for diagnostic information, there are still many obstacles such as short blood half-life, nonspecific biodistribution, rapid clearance, mild renal toxicity, and accumulation in the brain, as discussed recently [16].

MRI and Chemotherapy: A combination of nanoparticles with MRI contrast agents had a significant impact on the scientific world. Studies demonstrated and achieved promising results in terms of simultaneous diagnosis and treatment with MRI integration [16]. There are two different contrast agents classified based on magnetic property of the core of particles as T1 (longitudinal) and T2 (transverse) contrast agents, and for the T1 and T2 Weighted sequences of MRI, separate nanotheranostics are derived. Polymeric micelles are used as T1-weighted nanotheranostics. Drug-loaded micelles for cancer therapy were used as MRI contrast agents in pancreatic cancer. In this case, the poly (ethylene glycol)-poly (glutamic acid) block copolymer as imaging and treatment systems were used to form micelles that attract both Gd^{3+} and anticancer drug Oxaliplatin. MRI monitored the effect of treatment, signal development within the tumor, and changes in size . The micelles signals were up to seven times higher than the Gd-DTPA. The drug encapsulated with nanoteranostics led to a significant reduction in tumor volume and size. This study demonstrated, due to the excellent contrast resolution of MRI, that cancer can easily be distinguished from healthy tissue because it shows micelle deposition. This suggests that the dose of the chemotherapeutic drug can be rearranged while the tumor looks better [17].

In another study, Doxorubicin and gadolinium derivative (Gd-DOTA monoamine) were used in combination. Researches showed that C3d-lipo significantly improved therapeutic efficacy and toxicity when compared with free Doxorubicin. The therapeutic efficacy of the treatment was monitored by MRI [18, 19].

Recently, thermosensitive liposomes co-encapsulating Gd^{3+} and Doxorubicin have been tested *in vivo*. Rats used in preclinical studies were monitored by MRI to show the release and the uptake of Doxorubicin in locally heated tumors. A significant correlation was observed between the drug accumulation and the change of the T1 MRI relaxation time [20, 21].

Multifunctional magnetic nanohybrids are used as T2-weighted nanotheranostics. The effectiveness of this hybrid particle has been evaluated for theranostic purposes *in vivo* in a breast cancer model. The study showed a significant therapeutic efficiency compared to the use of free Doxorubicin [22]. Due to the toxicity of metal ions, negative contrast agents are based on magnetic iron oxide nanoparticles (SPIONs) and lead to a darker area in the T2-weighted image, thus are the most characteristic nanoparticle agents [23]. It is possible to increase the efficiency of MRI by coating many molecules with SPIONs [24]. For this purpose, recently, SPIONs have been widely used in cancer diagnosis and therapy, *via* magnetic targeting for example, because of their remarkable magnetic properties and chemical stabilities. Doxorubicin-loaded thermally cross-linked superparamagnetic iron oxide NPs (Dox@TCL-SPION) is another promising nanohybrid particles combining cancer diagnosis and therapy. This combination leads to simultaneous contrast imaging enhancement and antitumor therapy. Before injection of Dox@TCL-SPION, the tumor was hyperintense in T2-weighted MRI, while post-injection a significant darkening was observed, with a relative signal enhancement of 58%, suggesting considerable accumulation of the nanotheranostics [25 - 27]. Other functions may be added to drug carriers, such as imaging-controlled therapy, guidance, or heating (magnetic hyperthermia) by external magnetic fields. SPIONs can be used in a wide range of applications enabling in size, morphology, and functionalization. It is mainly used for the diagnosis of hepatic diseases and MR angiography. As compared to Gd, SPIONs have many advantages, including regulatable size, shape, surface modification, high sensitivity, and effectiveness at low concentrations due to their superparamagnetic features [20].

Photothermal Therapy with MRI; Photothermal therapy (PTT) is a therapy that kills apoptotic cells by heating them with Visible-NIR light. The increase in temperature ranges between 45°C and 300°C, and can be sufficiently effective. PTT only affects diseased tissues and causes minimal damage to healthy tissues. PTT and chemotherapy, known as Bimodal Therapy, can be performed by loading PLGA (poly (lactide-co-glycolide) nanotheranostics, which are taxol-loaded with iron oxide and conjugated to quantum points, to allow photothermal ablation of the tumor tissue. Alteration of the signal in the tumor area allows as contrast agent on MRI examination [28].

CT is another powerful diagnostic tool for imaging in terms of cost, performance, and availability and has become a necessary part of modern medicine today. Numerous advances have been revealed to make this technique more potent with improved signal sensitivity and rapid image acquisition and reconstruction. A significant disadvantage is that it works with an X-ray. However, the X-ray attenuation coefficient of different tissues in the body is different, based on this fact, CT can differentiate between soft tissues and bones to produce images for body structures [29]. CT images appear in grayscale, based on a decrease in the coefficients of different tissues in the body. The bone-like X-ray attenuating agent exhibits as light gray or white [30].

CT and Chemotherapy; Over the last years, there has been a significant increase in the improvement of nanoparticles as CT contrast agents [31]. Furthermore, nanoparticle loaded contrast agents include more contrast material and increased absorption of X-ray compared to standard iodine-based contrast agents, meaning that patients are exposed to less amount of X-ray doses [32]. A wide variety of compounds can be used as a contrast agent for coating nanoparticles. Nanoparticles have remarkable performances *in vivo* X-ray, especially CT angiography and tumor imaging according to studies. These nanohybrid materials are assumed to play a critical role in the expectation of medical diagnosis due to their ability to target specific biological markers, prolonged blood circulation, and described biologic clearances to display specific biological markers [4].

Ultrasound (US) is another imaging tool that is non-invasive, efficiently and safely applicable, and is a quickly accessed method today. When the contrast agent is administered, it causes a temporary increase in the permeability of the vessel walls and the accumulation of anticancer drugs in the surrounding cancerous tissues. This US-based imaging is performed with microbubble contrast agents [33].

US and Chemotherapy; Microbubble ultrasound contrast agents show very potent nanotheranostic tools for image-guided gene therapy applications. Although microbubble agents are typically used to enhance US contrast, they are becoming increasingly popular to target drugs systemically. In particular, Perfluorocarbon (PFC) NPs have received great interest for their application as a nanotheranostic system that combines ultrasound imaging using a contrast agent and provides a pharmacologically active agent. In the preclinical studies, a combination of US contrast agents and nanotheranostics has been used as chemotherapy, and promising results have been achieved [34, 35].

Interventional Imaging Practices: Interventional radiology applications are becoming very popular as a new diagnostic tool and at the same time therapy and nanotheranostics applications [36]. Interventional oncology includes a minimally invasive, real-time image-guided procedures and is generally associated with fewer complications, faster recovery times, shortened hospital stays, and lower costs compared with the conventional surgical procedures [37]. Interventional oncology allows for local drug delivery, vascular embolization, and direct ablation of tumors.

Interventional treatments delivered locally to damage cancerous tissues directly are associated with reduced infection rates, and quick recovery. Hospital stays are significantly reduced. Local-regional tumor ablation and embolization such as radiofrequency ablation, microwave ablation, cryoablation, transarterial chemoembolization (TACE) and/or radioembolization (TARE), and ultrasonography-guided delivery and therapy are becoming very popular. They have been reported as alternative treatment options for cancer patients. For instance, Yttrium-90 transarterial radioembolization (TARE) is a modern transcatheter locoregional therapy commonly used in primary and metastatic hepatic malignancies. It is one of the primary treatment modalities used in interventional oncology departments, and the frequency of utilization is increasing every day [38, 39]. These interventional procedures are used in combination with other drugs. Interventionally applied nanotherapeutics include enhancing anticancer activity by increasing tumor uptake of therapeutic agents, and thermal effects, thereby improving outcomes for patients. Transarterial embolization involves direct delivery of embolic agents loaded with nanoparticles to tumor vessels under real-time monitoring. This technique is expected to be more effective compared to TACE or TARE. These nanoparticles can provide the tumor with various combinations of cytotoxic agents, radionuclides, immune modulators. It can be used simultaneously with different tumor ablation techniques [40]. The limitation of the procedure is that if there is low blood flow, particles do not reach the cancerous tissue sufficiently. In this case, other interventional procedures, including chemotherapy, may be combined with nanoembolization to increase the blood perfusion and permeability to improve the penetration of nanotheranostic particles inside of tumors.

Optical Imaging: Optical imaging is one of the most common methods used in research. Optical imaging uses photons emitted by bioluminescence or fluorescent probes. The ability to detect low-energy photons apparent. It is more advantageous than other imaging methods because it does not expose the wide spectrum from light to near-infrared light, ionizing radiation, and has a high spatial resolution. Unfortunately, the disadvantage of this method is that deep tissues are not reached. Also, optical imaging has background artifacts, which is a significant problem. Choi *et al.* stated colon cancer using nanotheranostics with near-infrared fluorescent [41, 42].

Photoacoustic Imaging (PAI): In cancer control, PTT and PAI with nanotheranostics is mainly based on the combination of light and acoustic. It is a new hybrid imaging technology that can monitor internal body systems with very high speed and resolution. This method allows observing structures such as blood flow, lymph circulation, neuron synapses in a vivid manner. In the following years, the advantages of non-invasive imaging and the advantages of non-radiation in many subjects seem to be predicted such as in low-cost tomography. Non-invasive conversion of light energy to heat (PTT) or acoustic energy (PAI) has been extensively studied for cancer treatment and diagnosis using nanotheranostics [43].

When selecting the imaging method, the primary purpose should be considered, not just the contrast agent. For example, if a whole-body scan is required; MRI, CT, PET, and SPECT methods are recommended. However, rapid and low-cost organ-specific examinations, ultrasound can be performed. Moreover, optical and photoacoustic applications on the skin are the most appropriate to investigate superficial lesions such as peripheral joints (Table **1**) [44 - 46].

Advances in imaging technologies have resulted in additional consortium rules to standardize diagnostic imaging in oncology practiced today. Most notably, the Cheson criteria (1999, 2007, and 2014) have given instructions for the use of diagnostic imaging modalities [47, 48]. Besides, several other approaches have been introduced to assess different carcinomas accurately and the effects of immunotherapies on tumor responses [49 - 54]. The primary role of imaging in the treatment of oncology is emphasized. These criteria have become apparent that conventional anatomical imaging techniques, although very useful, have not supplied all the objective assessments needed to make accurate decisions.

Table 1. Overview of routinely used imaging modalities, advantages and disadvantages for the particular imaging method. (Baetke SC *et al*, Kunjachan *et al.* and Ehling *et al.*).

Imaging Method	Advantages	Disadvantages	Nanoparticulate Contrast Agents
MRI	High resolution	High costs	Gadolinium-containing probes
	High penetration	Low sensitivity	SPIONs
	Excellent soft tissue contrast	Time consuming	Paramagnetic polymers
	Variable options for structural, functional		ParaCEST agents
			Hyperpolarized probes
CT	High resolution	Insufficient soft tissue contrast without contrast agents	Iodine-based micelles and liposomes
	High penetration	Radiation exposure	Barium-based nanoparticles
	Good soft tissue contrast	Low sensitivity	Gold-based nanoparticles
	Low costs		Bismuth nanoparticles
	Fast imaging		
Ultrasound	High resolution	User dependence	Gas-filled microbubbles
	Easy accessible	Not appropriate for whole body imaging	Nanobubbles
	Real-time imaging		Air-releasing polymers
	Low costs		
	Fast imaging		
	Not X-ray		
Interventional Procedures	High resolution	No anatomical information	Local-regional tumor ablation
	Real-time imaging	Radiation exposure	Transarterial Embolization/ Chemoembolization/ Radioembolization
	More vascular information	High costs	Image-guided irreversible electroporation
		Minimally invasive method	Nanoelectroablation,
		Time consuming	RF ablation
			Microwave ablation
			Cryoablation

(Table 1) cont.....

Imaging Method	Advantages	Disadvantages	Nanoparticulate Contrast Agents
Optical Imaging	High sensitivity	Low penetration	Near-infrared fluorochrome-labeled nanoparticles
	The broad range of probes	High background signal	Quantum dots
	Low costs	Sensitive to artifacts	Fluorescent nanoparticle probes
Photoacoustic Imaging	High sensitivity	Limited penetration	Gold nanoparticles, gold nanorods
	Real-time imaging	Low specificity	Carbon nanotubes
	Low costs		Fluorescent/dye-loaded nanoparticles
PET	Very high sensitivity	Low resolution	Radioactive contrast agents
	Deep penetration	No anatomical information	Polymeric nanoparticles
	Quantitative analyses	Radiation exposure	
		High costs	
Single Photon Emission CT	Very high sensitivity	Low resolution	Technetium-labelled gold nanoparticles
	High penetration	No anatomical information	Indium-labeled liposomes
	Long-circulating radionuclides	Radioactive	Nano and microcolloids
		High cost	

Researchers have shown great interest in developing methods for evaluating data from CT and MRI studies. Image analysis help shape new areas of radiological imaging to assess the relationship between CT and MRI and molecular biology of tumors [12].

Nuclear Medicine Applications

Nuclear imaging allowed much earlier diagnosis and treatment, and better prognosis has opened a new door to non-invasively *in vitro/ex vivo* assessment in the oncology field and for personalized medicine [7].

Single Photon Emission Computed Tomography and Positron Emission Tomography (SPECT and PET) Imaging: Nuclear medicine imaging techniques, including single-photon emission computed tomography (SPECT) and positron emission tomography (PET) have been commonly used for diagnosis and treatment of cancers. PET and SPECT imaging need the use of a radionuclide that is injected into the patient. Using scanner detectors that encircle or revolving around a patient, two- or three-dimensional images of radioactivity distribution within the body are obtained [7].

By the application of nanotechnology in nuclear medicine, it has been possible to make the diagnosis and treatment of diseases simultaneously as non-invasive and real-time in one nano-sized drug delivery system. A nanotheranostic probe for nuclear medicine gives combined diagnostic and therapeutic capabilities by different radiolabeling emitters (α, β^+, β^-, γ) used for imaging and/or therapy [55]. The radiolabeled nanoparticles consist of the labeling of radionuclides onto the nanomaterials that cause deeper penetration increasing internal radiotherapy in cancer cells and inducing cell death [56].

An ideal radionuclide nanotheranostic probe has properties such as long shelf life, easily accessible radionuclides, convenient half-life, easy and high marking efficiency, *in vivo* stability, lack of immunological reaction, rapidly clearance from circulation and directed to the target, high image quality, retention of radionuclide in liposome and non-toxic metabolites [57]. Although various inorganic nanoparticles (micelles, microbubbles, dendrimers, liposomes and other polymeric structures) are possible labeling with radionuclide marking technique, in terms of physicochemical properties of passive and active targeting content, the most suitable storage units are liposomes [58]. Liposomes, spherical vesicles of lipid bilayers (100–800nm in diameter) are commonly used nanoparticles for internal radiotherapy of cancer [59]. The studies revealed, liposome systems have a specific influence on the absorbed doses in tumor cells. Also, multifunctional nanoparticle PET agents for tumor targeting and drug loading have been developed [60].

In vivo stability is essential in radionuclide labeling. Because, free radioactive agent, accumulates in non-target organs, such as thyroid, stomach, and kidney, and quality of imaging and therapy is decreased. Chelating agents such as diethylenetriamine penta-acetic acid (DTPA) and hekzametil-propilen-aminoksim (HMPAO), including reducing agent glutathione, are used to increase *in vivo* stability [61].

The Commonly Used Therapeutic Radionuclides for Labeling Nanoparticles

1. α-particle Emitters

The therapeutic radionuclide α-particle emitters with energies between 4-8 MeV show very high linear energy transfer (LET, ~100 keV/μm), which can emerge severe cytotoxicity with direct DNA damage, but their ejection range is quite short (40–80μm) and equivalent to a few cell layers. Therefore, the healthy cells around the cancer cells are less affected. α-particle therapy reduces or treats the tumor even in patients who are radiation-resistant or have not benefited from other treatments.

Alpha-emitting radionuclides used for nanoparticle labeling are Terbium-149 ([149]Tb), Astatine-211 ([211]At), Bismuth-212 ([212]Bi), Bi-213 ([213]Bi), Radium-223 ([223]Ra), Actinium-225 ([225]Ac), and Thorium-227 ([227]Th) [62]. In one study, α-emitter-loaded sterically stabilized liposomes were conjugated to a folate-F(ab′)2 construct for tumor-targeted radiotherapy [63]. Another study investigated the different factors on the retention of both [225]Ac (up to ~ 90% in 30 days) and its daughter nuclei [213]Bi within the liposomes [64]. [225]Ac (half-life 10days) is an α-emitting radioisotope. Radiolabeling prostate-specific membrane antigen (PSMA)-617 with α-emitting [225]Ac shows an effective response in patients with metastatic castration-resistant prostate cancer [65]. PSMA-617 is a theranostic probe that can be applied both for imaging and therapy. In clinical practice, PSMA-11 is often used for diagnostic staging, and the dodecanetetraacetic acid (DOTA)- analog PSMA-617 is used for treatment [66].

[211]At-loaded liposomes were investigated for various tumor-targeted radiotherapy. Trastuzumab-modified gold nanoparticles labeled with [211]At has been found as a potential radiobioconjugate for local treatment of human epidermal growth factor receptor (HER)2 -positive breast cancer [67, 68]. Recently, the results of one study demonstrated that [149]Tb and [161]Tb-PSMA-617 have suitable decay characteristics for an effective treatment of prostate cancer patients [69].

Other agents are [213]Bi, which decays upon α- and β-particle emission and [223]Ra (half-life 11.4 days), which is used in clinical routine as [223]Ra -RaCl2 (Xofigo®) for the treatment of prostate cancer-related bone metastases [70, 71].

2. β-particle Emitters

β-particle emitters (range between 1 and 10mm with energies between 0.1 and 1 MeV) are the most commonly used radionuclides in cancer therapy. These radioisotopes released β-particles (*i.e.* electrons) that interact with atoms. They have lower energy and cause lower cytotoxicity, but can travel longer distances in the circulation and kill tumor cells by indirect damage to the DNA [72]. The most commonly used radionuclides are ^{131}I, ^{177}Lu, ^{90}Y, [67]Cu, [186/188]Re, [198]Au. 131I radioiodine (90% beta minus emission with a low tissue penetration of 0.4 mm; half-life eight days) commonly used for the treatment of thyroid cancer is both therapeutic and diagnostic agents. There are several studies used [131]I- labeled nanoparticles, including ^{131}I-labeled dextran-coated magnetic nanoparticles and conjugated with an anti-VEGF monoclonal antibody; radioiodine labeled liposomes, integrin αvβ3-targeted radiotherapy, pre-targeted immunotherapy [73].

[131]I was seen to be quite efficient in labeling liposomes [74, 75]. [90]Y (tissue penetration 2.5mm) is a pure beta minus emitter and has an optimal decay half-life (2.7 days) and a more extended range in tissue [76]. Investigation of ^{90}Y-labeled liposomes revealed that it has suitable properties for radioimmunotherapy, internal radiotherapy, and targeting tumor angiogenesis [77]. Selective internal radiation therapy (SIRT) or transarterial radio embolization (TARE) applied ^{90}Y microspheres are widely used in primary or metastatic liver tumors. Recently, SIRT combined chemotherapeutics is a research topic, and combined therapy is thought to be more efficacious [78].

Lutetium-177 (^{177}Lu) (long half-life 6.7 days) emits low β^- energy (Eβmax = 497.1 keV) and has been commonly used in peptide radionuclide therapy. [177]Lu has approximately 2mm tissue penetration, which is suitable for treating small tumor cells and micrometastases [79]. The gold nanoparticles radiolabeled with ^{177}Lu and conjugated to RGD (-Arg-Gly-Asp-), Lys3-Bombesin, and Tat [49-57] peptides have been developed for molecular imaging and internal radiotherapy [80]. In another study, PEG-coated [177]Lu -DOTATATE-PLGA-nanoparticles (PEG- LuD-NP) were used for somatostatin receptor (SSR) positive tumors. The nanocarrier-mediated-PRRT was revealed that reduced renal radiation dose and cytotoxicity associated with conventional PRRT [81]. Recently, [177]Lu -gold nanoparticles (AuNPs) conjugated to different peptides (RGD (-Arg-Gly-Asp-), Lys3-Bombesin, and Tat [49 - 57] used simultaneously as molecular imaging agents, radiotherapy and thermal-ablation systems were developed for cancer treatment and drug delivery systems [80]. Multiradioisotope labeling with a dual-energy combined internal therapy using ^{177}Lu together with ^{90}Y in one particle can have an effect on therapeutic outcome [82].

[188]Re (half-life: 17h) emits beta minus particles (25.6%) and gamma rays for imaging (15.1%) [83]. [188]Re-loaded glutathione-encapsulated liposomes were investigated for nanoparticle-based radiotherapy. The studies showed well *in vivo* stability and feasibility of using liposomes for internal radiotherapy because of reduced absorbed dose in normal tissue [84]. A dosimetric analysis report evaluated radionuclides ([188]Re- liposomes) or combination of radionuclides and chemotherapeutic drugs ([188]Re-doxorubicin-liposomes, termed "[188]Re-DXR-liposome") for treating colon carcinoma, has been found these nanoparticles were feasible and efficacious for cancer therapy [85]. Furthermore, the silica-coated magnetite nanoparticles and superparamagnetic iron oxide nanoparticles labeled with [188]Re have been designed for magnetically targeted radiotherapy [86, 87]. [89]Zr has a half-life of several days that is optimal for *in vivo* imaging of macromolecules and nano-sized structures and is suitable for the biological half-life and pharmacokinetics of immunoconjugates. [89]Zr-labeled carbon nanotubes are used for the treatment of tumor vasculature [88]. This radionuclide has low

positron energy of 356 keV that results in high-resolution PET images. Additionally, ^{89}Zr and ^{90}Y provide an efficient combination of radioimmunotherapies.

The theranostic pair of Copper-64 (^{64}Cu;19% β$^+$, 38% β$^-$) and Copper -67 (^{67}Cu; β$^-$, γ) is used both in diagnostic and radiotherapeutic research [90]. ^{67}Cu has the most prolonged half-life (2.6 days) copper radioisotope and emits β$^-$ (beta) particles and γ rays. It is suitable for both imaging and radiotherapy. The application of different ^{67}Cu-labeled antibodies, magnetic nanoparticles, gold nanoparticles, and inorganic quantum dots and copper sulfide nanoparticles are investigated for nanotheranostics [89, 90]. Also, ^{64}Cu - labeled nanoparticles have been used imaging and combined radiotherapy, chemotherapy, and photothermal therapy, which is highly superior to any of the single therapeutic modalities [91, 92]. Furthermore, the multifunctional nanoparticles (^{68}Ga/^{64}Cu and ^{177}Lu) or dual-energy combined internal therapy using (^{177}Lu and ^{90}Y) dual radioisotope tagging can be used for multiradioisotope labeling or a multitargeting strategy (prostate-specific membrane antigen (PSMA), Arg-Gly- Asp (RGD), and ^{64}Cu for effective biologic dose (BED) prediction and confirmation, and ^{177}Lu for radionuclide therapy) [56].

3. Auger Electron Emitters

Auger electron-emitting radioisotopes like Indium-111 (^{111}In) have short-ranges (<1 μm), and are generally not suitable for nanoparticle-based radiotherapy. But Auger electrons have a high energy loss over a very short distance with the lowest possible side effect [56, 57].

Vascular endothelial growth factor receptor (VEGF-R), epidermal growth factor (EGFR), and αvβ3 integrin have an essential role in tumor growth and angiogenesis. In several studies, ^{111}In-labeled VEGF-R, EGFR, αvβ3 integrin, and monoclonal antibody nanoparticles have been used in imaging and therapy of cancer [93].

CONCLUDING REMARKS

With the emergence of the nanotheranostic concept used in cancer patients has demonstrated the importance of multidisciplinary approaches which need to be improved. Simultaneous imaging and diagnosis have been very exciting. With future nanotechnology and newly developed agents, it can offer the best possible monitoring and personalized treatment plans for cancer patients. However, nanotherapeutics will guarantee the success of cancer treatment in the coming years if the most appropriate treatment is administered to the right patients, who are appropriately selected. It is believed that the development of nanoteranostics can change the way cancer is diagnosed, followed-up, and treated.

CONSENT FOR PUBLICATION

Not applicable.

CONFLICT OF INTEREST

The authors confirm that the contents of this chapter have no conflict of interest.

ACKNOWLEDGEMENTS

Declared none.

REFERENCES

[1]   Sager S, Akgün E, Uslu-Beşli L, *et al.* Comparison of PERCIST and RECIST criteria for evaluation of therapy response after yttrium-90 microsphere therapy in patients with hepatocellular carcinoma and those with metastatic colorectal carcinoma. Nucl Med Commun 2019; 40(5): 461-8.
        [http://dx.doi.org/10.1097/MNM.0000000000001014] [PMID: 30896544]

[2]   Kiessling F, Mertens ME, Grimm J, Lammers T. Nanoparticles for imaging: top or flop? Radiology 2014; 273(1): 10-28.
        [http://dx.doi.org/10.1148/radiol.14131520] [PMID: 25247562]

[3]   Chen H, Zhang W, Zhu G, Xie J, Chen X. Rethinking cancer nanotheranostics. Nat Rev Mater 2017; 2: 17024.
        [http://dx.doi.org/10.1038/natrevmats.2017.24] [PMID: 29075517]

[4]   Pan D, Schirra CO, Wickline SA, Lanza GM. Multicolor computed tomographic molecular imaging with noncrystalline high-metal-density nanobeacons. Contrast Media Mol Imaging 2014; 9(1): 13-25.
        [http://dx.doi.org/10.1002/cmmi.1571] [PMID: 24470291]

[5]   Mura S, Couvreur P. Nanotheranostics for personalized medicine. Adv Drug Deliv Rev 2012; 64(13): 1394-416.
        [http://dx.doi.org/10.1016/j.addr.2012.06.006] [PMID: 22728642]

[6]   Blau R, Krivitsky A, Epshtein Y, Satchi-Fainaro R. Are nanotheranostics and nanodiagnostics-guided drug delivery stepping stones towards precision medicine? Drug Resist Updat 2016; 27: 39-58.
        [http://dx.doi.org/10.1016/j.drup.2016.06.003] [PMID: 27449597]

[7]   Sumer B, Gao J. Theranostic nanomedicine for cancer. Nanomedicine (Lond) 2008; 3(2): 137-40.
        [http://dx.doi.org/10.2217/17435889.3.2.137] [PMID: 18373419]

[8]   Weissleder R, Schwaiger MC, Gambhir SS, Hricak H. Imaging approaches to optimize molecular therapies. Sci Transl Med 2016; 8(355): 355-16.
        [http://dx.doi.org/10.1126/scitranslmed.aaf3936] [PMID: 27605550]

[9]   Di Sanzo M, Cipolloni L, Borro M, *et al.* Clinical applications of personalized medicine: a new paradigm and challenge. Curr Pharm Biotechnol 2017; 18(3): 194-203.
        [http://dx.doi.org/10.2174/1389201018666170224105600] [PMID: 28240172]

[10]   Maughan T. The promise and the hype of 'personalised medicine. New Bioeth 2017; 23(1): 13-20.
        [http://dx.doi.org/10.1080/20502877.2017.1314886] [PMID: 28517988]

[11]   Wu B, Lu ST, Yu H, *et al.* Gadolinium-chelate functionalized bismuth nanotheranostic agent for *in vivo* MRI/CT/PAI imaging-guided photothermal cancer therapy. Biomaterials 2018; 159: 37-47.

[http://dx.doi.org/10.1016/j.biomaterials.2017.12.022] [PMID: 29309992]

[12] Van Heertum RL, Scarimbolo R, Ford R, Berdougo E, O'Neal M. Companion diagnostics and molecular imaging-enhanced approaches for oncology clinical trials. Drug Des Devel Ther 2015; 9: 5215-23.
[http://dx.doi.org/10.2147/DDDT.S87561] [PMID: 26392755]

[13] Miller AB, Hoogstraten B, Staquet M, Winkler A. Reporting results of cancer treatment. Cancer 1981; 47(1): 207-14.
[http://dx.doi.org/10.1002/1097-0142(19810101)47:1<207::AID-CNCR2820470134>3.0.CO;2-6]
[PMID: 7459811]

[14] Weinstein JS, Varallyay CG, Dosa E, *et al.* Superparamagnetic iron oxide nanoparticles: diagnostic magnetic resonance imaging and potential therapeutic applications in neurooncology and central nervous system inflammatory pathologies, a review. J Cereb Blood Flow Metab 2010; 30(1): 15-35.
[http://dx.doi.org/10.1038/jcbfm.2009.192] [PMID: 19756021]

[15] Yang W, Guo W, Le W, *et al.* Albumin-Bioinspired Gd: CuS nanotheranostic agent for *in vivo* photoacoustic/magnetic resonance imaging-guided tumor-targeted photothermal therapy. ACS Nano 2016; 10(11): 10245-57.
[http://dx.doi.org/10.1021/acsnano.6b05760] [PMID: 27791364]

[16] Harisinghani MG, Barentsz J, Hahn PF, *et al.* Noninvasive detection of clinically occult lymph-node metastases in prostate cancer. N Engl J Med 2003; 348(25): 2491-9.
[http://dx.doi.org/10.1056/NEJMoa022749] [PMID: 12815134]

[17] Weissleder R, Pittet MJ. Imaging in the era of molecular oncology. Nature 2008; 452(7187): 580-9.
[http://dx.doi.org/10.1038/nature06917] [PMID: 18385732]

[18] Lee SY, Jeon SI, Jung S, Chung IJ, Ahn CH. Targeted multimodal imaging modalities. Adv Drug Deliv Rev 2014; 76: 60-78.
[http://dx.doi.org/10.1016/j.addr.2014.07.009] [PMID: 25064554]

[19] Ramalho J, Ramalho M. Gadolinium deposition and chronic toxicity. Magn Reson Imaging Clin N Am 2017; 25(4): 765-78.
[http://dx.doi.org/10.1016/j.mric.2017.06.007] [PMID: 28964466]

[20] Naseri N, Ajorlou E, Asghari F, Pilehvar-Soltanahmadi Y. An update on nanoparticle-based contrast agents in medical imaging. Artif Cells Nanomed Biotechnol 2018; 46(6): 1111-21.
[http://dx.doi.org/10.1080/21691401.2017.1379014] [PMID: 28933183]

[21] Song R, Zhang M, Liu Y, *et al.* A multifunctional nanotheranostic for the intelligent MRI diagnosis and synergistic treatment of hypoxic tumor. Biomaterials 2018; 175: 123-33.
[http://dx.doi.org/10.1016/j.biomaterials.2018.05.018] [PMID: 29804000]

[22] Na HB, Song IC, Hyeon T. Inorganic nanoparticles for MRI contrast agents. Adv Mater 2009; 21: 2133-48.
[http://dx.doi.org/10.1002/adma.200802366]

[23] Fang C, Zhang M. Multifunctional magnetic nanoparticles for medical imaging applications. J Mater Chem 2009; 19: 6258-66.
[http://dx.doi.org/10.1039/b902182e] [PMID: 20593005]

[24] Khalkhali M, Rostamizadeh K, Sadighian S, Khoeini F, Naghibi M, Hamidi M. The impact of polymer coatings on magnetite nanoparticles performance as MRI contrast agents: a comparative study. Daru 2015; 23: 45.
[http://dx.doi.org/10.1186/s40199-015-0124-7] [PMID: 26381740]

[25] Kandasamy G, Maity D. Recent advances in superparamagnetic iron oxide nanoparticles (SPIONs) for *in vitro* and *in vivo* cancer nanotheranostics. Int J Pharm 2015; 496(2): 191-218.
[http://dx.doi.org/10.1016/j.ijpharm.2015.10.058] [PMID: 26520409]

[26] Mahmoudi M, Sant S, Wang B, Laurent S, Sen T. Superparamagnetic iron oxide nanoparticles

(SPIONs): development, surface modification and applications in chemotherapy. Adv Drug Deliv Rev 2011; 63(1-2): 24-46.
[http://dx.doi.org/10.1016/j.addr.2010.05.006] [PMID: 20685224]

[27]   Revia RA, Zhang M. Magnetite nanoparticles for cancer diagnosis, treatment, and treatment monitoring: recent advances. Mater Today (Kidlington) 2016; 19(3): 157-68.
[http://dx.doi.org/10.1016/j.mattod.2015.08.022] [PMID: 27524934]

[28]   Santhosh PB, Ulrih NP. Multifunctional superparamagnetic iron oxide nanoparticles: promising tools in cancer theranostics. Cancer Lett 2013; 336(1): 8-17.
[http://dx.doi.org/10.1016/j.canlet.2013.04.032] [PMID: 23664890]

[29]   Popovtzer R, Agrawal A, Kotov NA, *et al.* Targeted gold nanoparticles enable molecular CT imaging of cancer. Nano Lett 2008; 8(12): 4593-6.
[http://dx.doi.org/10.1021/nl8029114] [PMID: 19367807]

[30]   Cormode DP, Naha PC, Fayad ZA. Nanoparticle contrast agents for computed tomography: a focus on micelles. Contrast Media Mol Imaging 2014; 9(1): 37-52.
[http://dx.doi.org/10.1002/cmmi.1551] [PMID: 24470293]

[31]   He W, Ai K, Lu L. Nanoparticulate X-ray CT contrast agents. Sci China Chem 2015; 58: 753-60.
[http://dx.doi.org/10.1007/s11426-015-5351-8]

[32]   Mukundan S Jr, Ghaghada KB, Badea CT, *et al.* A liposomal nanoscale contrast agent for preclinical CT in mice. AJR Am J Roentgenol 2006; 186(2): 300-7.
[http://dx.doi.org/10.2214/AJR.05.0523] [PMID: 16423931]

[33]   Xiong F, Nirupama S, Sirsi SR, Lacko A, Hoyt K. Ultrasound-stimulated drug delivery using therapeutic reconstituted high-density lipoprotein nanoparticles. Nanotheranostics 2017; 1(4): 440-9.
[http://dx.doi.org/10.7150/ntno.21905] [PMID: 29188177]

[34]   Sorace AG, Saini R, Rosenthal E, Warram JM, Zinn KR, Hoyt K. Optical fluorescent imaging to monitor temporal effects of microbubble-mediated ultrasound therapy. IEEE Trans Ultrason Ferroelectr Freq Control 2013; 60(2): 281-9.
[http://dx.doi.org/10.1109/TUFFC.2013.2564] [PMID: 23357902]

[35]   Sirsi SR, Borden MA. Advances in ultrasound mediated gene therapy using microbubble contrast agents. Theranostics 2012; 2(12): 1208-22.
[http://dx.doi.org/10.7150/thno.4306] [PMID: 23382777]

[36]   Parchur AK, Sharma G, Jagtap JM, *et al.* Vascular interventional radiology-guided photothermal therapy of colorectal cancer liver metastasis with theranostic gold nanorods. ACS Nano 2018; 12(7): 6597-611.
[http://dx.doi.org/10.1021/acsnano.8b01424] [PMID: 29969226]

[37]   Baum RA, Baum S. Interventional radiology: a half century of innovation. Radiology 2014; 273(2) (Suppl.): S75-91.
[http://dx.doi.org/10.1148/radiol.14140534] [PMID: 25340439]

[38]   Li J, Liu F, Gupta S, Li C. Interventional nanotheranostics of pancreatic ductal adenocarcinoma. Theranostics 2016; 6(9): 1393-402.
[http://dx.doi.org/10.7150/thno.15122] [PMID: 27375787]

[39]   Brown DB, Narayanan G. Interventional radiology and the pancreatic cancer patient. Cancer J 2012; 18(6): 591-601.
[http://dx.doi.org/10.1097/PPO.0b013e3182745bee] [PMID: 23187847]

[40]   Murata S, Mine T, Sugihara F, *et al.* Interventional treatment for unresectable hepatocellular carcinoma. World J Gastroenterol 2014; 20(37): 13453-65.
[http://dx.doi.org/10.3748/wjg.v20.i37.13453] [PMID: 25309076]

[41]   Song J, Yang X, Yang Z, *et al.* Rational design of branched nanoporous gold nanoshells with enhanced physico-optical properties for optical imaging and cancer therapy. ACS Nano 2017; 11(6):

6102-13.
[http://dx.doi.org/10.1021/acsnano.7b02048] [PMID: 28605594]

[42]   Choi KY, Jeon EJ, Yoon HY, *et al.* Theranostic nanoparticles based on PEGylated hyaluronic acid for the diagnosis, therapy and monitoring of colon cancer. Biomaterials 2012; 33(26): 6186-93.
[http://dx.doi.org/10.1016/j.biomaterials.2012.05.029] [PMID: 22687759]

[43]   Yang Z, Song J, Tang W, *et al.* Stimuli-responsive nanotheranostics for real-time monitoring drug release by photoacoustic imaging. Theranostics 2019; 9(2): 526-36.
[http://dx.doi.org/10.7150/thno.30779] [PMID: 30809290]

[44]   Baetke SC, Lammers T, Kiessling F. Applications of nanoparticles for diagnosis and therapy of cancer. Br J Radiol 2015; 88(1054): 20150207.
[http://dx.doi.org/10.1259/bjr.20150207] [PMID: 25969868]

[45]   Kunjachan S, Jayapaul J, Mertens ME, Storm G, Kiessling F, Lammers T. Theranostic systems and strategies for monitoring nanomedicine-mediated drug targeting. Curr Pharm Biotechnol 2012; 13(4): 609-22.
[http://dx.doi.org/10.2174/138920112799436302] [PMID: 22214503]

[46]   Ehling J, Lammers T, Kiessling F. Non-invasive imaging for studying anti-angiogenic therapy effects. Thromb Haemost 2013; 109(3): 375-90.
[http://dx.doi.org/10.1160/TH12-10-0721] [PMID: 23407722]

[47]   Cheson BD, Pfistner B, Juweid ME, *et al.* Revised response criteria for malignant lymphoma. J Clin Oncol 2007; 25(5): 579-86.
[http://dx.doi.org/10.1200/JCO.2006.09.2403] [PMID: 17242396]

[48]   Fournier L, Ammari S, Thiam R, Cuénod CA. Imaging criteria for assessing tumour response: RECIST, mRECIST, Cheson. Diagn Interv Imaging 2014; 95(7-8): 689-703.
[http://dx.doi.org/10.1016/j.diii.2014.05.002] [PMID: 24951349]

[49]   Cheson BD, Greenberg PL, Bennett JM, *et al.* Clinical application and proposal for modification of the International Working Group (IWG) response criteria in myelodysplasia. Blood 2006; 108(2): 419-25.
[http://dx.doi.org/10.1182/blood-2005-10-4149] [PMID: 16609072]

[50]   Scher HI, Halabi S, Tannock I, *et al.* Design and end points of clinical trials for patients with progressive prostate cancer and castrate levels of testosterone: recommendations of the Prostate Cancer Clinical Trials Working Group. J Clin Oncol 2008; 26(7): 1148-59.
[http://dx.doi.org/10.1200/JCO.2007.12.4487] [PMID: 18309951]

[51]   Wolchok JD, Hoos A, O'Day S, *et al.* Guidelines for the evaluation of immune therapy activity in solid tumors: immune-related response criteria. Clin Cancer Res 2009; 15(23): 7412-20.
[http://dx.doi.org/10.1158/1078-0432.CCR-09-1624] [PMID: 19934295]

[52]   Cheson BD, Bennett JM, Kopecky KJ, *et al.* Revised recommendations of the international working group for diagnosis, standardization of response criteria, treatment outcomes, and reporting standards for therapeutic trials in acute myeloid leukemia. J Clin Oncol 2003; 21(24): 4642-9.
[http://dx.doi.org/10.1200/JCO.2003.04.036] [PMID: 14673054]

[53]   Lencioni R, Llovet JM. Modified RECIST (mRECIST) assessment for hepatocellular carcinoma. Semin Liver Dis 2010; 30(1): 52-60.
[http://dx.doi.org/10.1055/s-0030-1247132] [PMID: 20175033]

[54]   van den Bent MJ, Wefel JS, Schiff D, *et al.* Response assessment in neuro-oncology (a report of the RANO group): assessment of outcome in trials of diffuse low-grade gliomas. Lancet Oncol 2011; 12(6): 583-93.
[http://dx.doi.org/10.1016/S1470-2045(11)70057-2] [PMID: 21474379]

[55]   Drude N, Tienken L, Mottaghy FM. Theranostic and nanotheranostic probes in nuclear medicine. Methods 2017; 130: 14-22.
[http://dx.doi.org/10.1016/j.ymeth.2017.07.004] [PMID: 28698069]

[56]   Lee YS, Kim YI, Lee DS. Future perspectives of radionanomedicine using the novel micelle-encapsulation method for surface modification. Nucl Med Mol Imaging 2015; 49(3): 170-3.
[http://dx.doi.org/10.1007/s13139-015-0358-9] [PMID: 26279689]

[57]   Hong H, Zhang Y, Sun J, Cai W. Molecular imaging and therapy of cancer with radiolabeled nanoparticles. Nano Today 2009; 4(5): 399-413.
[http://dx.doi.org/10.1016/j.nantod.2009.07.001] [PMID: 20161038]

[58]   Silindir M, Erdoğan S, Özer AY, Maia S. Liposomes and their applications in molecular imaging. J Drug Target 2012; 20(5): 401-15.
[http://dx.doi.org/10.3109/1061186X.2012.685477] [PMID: 22553977]

[59]   Torchilin VP. Recent advances with liposomes as pharmaceutical carriers. Nat Rev Drug Discov 2005; 4(2): 145-60.
[http://dx.doi.org/10.1038/nrd1632] [PMID: 15688077]

[60]   Xiao Y, Hong H, Javadi A, *et al.* Multifunctional unimolecular micelles for cancer-targeted drug delivery and positron emission tomography imaging. Biomaterials 2012; 33(11): 3071-82.
[http://dx.doi.org/10.1016/j.biomaterials.2011.12.030] [PMID: 22281424]

[61]   Laverman P, Boerman OC, Storm G. Radiolabeling of liposomes for scintigraphic imaging. Methods Enzymol 2003; 373: 234-48.
[http://dx.doi.org/10.1016/S0076-6879(03)73015-8] [PMID: 14714407]

[62]   Seo Y. Quantitative imaging of alpha-emitting therapeutic radiopharmaceuticals. Nucl Med Mol Imaging 2019; 53(3): 182-8.
[http://dx.doi.org/10.1007/s13139-019-00589-8] [PMID: 31231438]

[63]   Henriksen G, Schoultz BW, Michaelsen TE, Bruland ØS, Larsen RH. Sterically stabilized liposomes as a carrier for alpha-emitting radium and actinium radionuclides. Nucl Med Biol 2004; 31(4): 441-9.
[http://dx.doi.org/10.1016/j.nucmedbio.2003.11.004] [PMID: 15093814]

[64]   Sofou S, Thomas JL, Lin HY, McDevitt MR, Scheinberg DA, Sgouros G. Engineered liposomes for potential alpha-particle therapy of metastatic cancer. J Nucl Med 2004; 45(2): 253-60.
[PMID: 14960644]

[65]   Sathekge M, Bruchertseifer F, Vorster M, *et al.* A predictors of overall and disease free survival in metastatic castration-resistant prostate cancer patients receiving [225]Ac-PSMA-617 radioligand therapy. J Nucl Med 2019. May 17.
[http://dx.doi.org/10.2967/jnumed.119.229229] [PMID: 31101746]

[66]   Bouchelouche K, Turkbey B, Choyke PL. PSMA PET and radionuclide therapy in prostate cancer. Semin Nucl Med 2016; 46(6): 522-35.
[http://dx.doi.org/10.1053/j.semnuclmed.2016.07.006] [PMID: 27825432]

[67]   Dziawer Ł, Majkowska-Pilip A, Gaweł D, *et al.* Trastuzumab-modified gold nanoparticles labeled with [211]At as a prospective tool for local treatment of HER2-positive breast cancer. Nanomaterials (Basel) 2019; 9(4): E632.
[http://dx.doi.org/10.3390/nano9040632] [PMID: 31003512]

[68]   Ohshima Y, Kono N, Yokota Y, *et al.* Anti-tumor effects and potential therapeutic response biomarkers in α-emitting *meta*-[211]At-astato-benzylguanidine therapy for malignant pheochromocytoma explored by RNA-sequencing. Theranostics 2019; 9(6): 1538-49.
[http://dx.doi.org/10.7150/thno.30353] [PMID: 31037122]

[69]   Müller C, Singh A, Umbricht CA, *et al.* Preclinical investigations and first-in-human application of [152]Tb-PSMA-617 for PET/CT imaging of prostate cancer. EJNMMI Res 2019; 9(1): 68.
[http://dx.doi.org/10.1186/s13550-019-0538-1] [PMID: 31346796]

[70]   McDevitt MR, Scheinberg DA. Ac-225 and her daughters: the many faces of Shiva. Cell Death Differ 2002; 9(6): 593-4.
[http://dx.doi.org/10.1038/sj.cdd.4401047] [PMID: 12032666]

[71]   Parker C, Nilsson S, Heinrich D, *et al.* Alpha emitter radium-223 and survival in metastatic prostate cancer. N Engl J Med 2013; 369(3): 213-23.
[http://dx.doi.org/10.1056/NEJMoa1213755] [PMID: 23863050]

[72]   Qaim SM, Spahn I. Development of novel radionuclides for medical applications. J Labelled Comp Radiopharm 2018; 61(3): 126-40.
[http://dx.doi.org/10.1002/jlcr.3578] [PMID: 29110328]

[73]   Chen J, Wu H, Han D, Xie C. Using anti-VEGF McAb and magnetic nanoparticles as double-targeting vector for the radioimmunotherapy of liver cancer. Cancer Lett 2006; 231(2): 169-75.
[http://dx.doi.org/10.1016/j.canlet.2005.01.024] [PMID: 16399221]

[74]   Kostarelos K, Emfietzoglou D. Tissue dosimetry of liposome-radionuclide complexes for internal radiotherapy: toward liposome-targeted therapeutic radiopharmaceuticals. Anticancer Res 2000; 20(5A): 3339-45.
[PMID: 11062762]

[75]   Mougin-Degraef M, Bourdeau C, Jestin E, *et al.* Doubly radiolabeled liposomes for pretargeted radioimmunotherapy. Int J Pharm 2007; 344(1-2): 110-7.
[http://dx.doi.org/10.1016/j.ijpharm.2007.05.024] [PMID: 17592745]

[76]   Stein R, Chen S, Haim S, Goldenberg DM. Advantage of yttrium-90-labeled over iodine-131-labeled monoclonal antibodies in the treatment of a human lung carcinoma xenograft. Cancer 1997; 80(12) (Suppl.): 2636-41.
[http://dx.doi.org/10.1002/(SICI)1097-0142(19971215)80:12+<2636::AID-CNCR39>3.0.CO;2-B] [PMID: 9406718]

[77]   Li L, Wartchow CA, Danthi SN, *et al.* A novel antiangiogenesis therapy using an integrin antagonist or anti-Flk-1 antibody coated ^{90}Y-labeled nanoparticles. Int J Radiat Oncol Biol Phys 2004; 58(4): 1215-27.
[http://dx.doi.org/10.1016/j.ijrobp.2003.10.057] [PMID: 15001266]

[78]   Kennedy A, Brown DB, Feilchenfeldt J, *et al.* Safety of selective internal radiation therapy (SIRT) with yttrium-90 microspheres combined with systemic anticancer agents: expert consensus. J Gastrointest Oncol 2017; 8(6): 1079-99.
[http://dx.doi.org/10.21037/jgo.2017.09.10] [PMID: 29299370]

[79]   Baum RP, Kulkarni HR. THERANOSTICS: From molecular imaging using Ga-68 labeled tracers and PET/CT to personalized radionuclide therapy- the bad berka experience. Theranostics 2012; 2(5): 437-47.
[http://dx.doi.org/10.7150/thno.3645] [PMID: 22768024]

[80]   Ferro-Flores G, Ocampo-García BE, Santos-Cuevas CL, de María Ramírez F, Azorín-Vega EP, Meléndez-Alafort L. Theranostic radiopharmaceuticals based on gold nanoparticles labeled with ^{177}Lu and conjugated to peptides. Curr Radiopharm 2015; 8(2): 150-9.
[http://dx.doi.org/10.2174/1874471008666150313115423] [PMID: 25771363]

[81]   Arora G, Dubey P, Shukla J, Ghosh S, Bandopadhyaya G. Evaluation of cytotoxic and tumor targeting capability of ^{177}Lu-DOTATATE-nanoparticles: a trailblazing strategy in peptide receptor radionuclide therapy. Ann Nucl Med 2016; 30(5): 334-45.
[http://dx.doi.org/10.1007/s12149-016-1067-x] [PMID: 26897009]

[82]   de Jong MI. Breeman WA, Valkema R, Bernard BF, Krenning EP. Combination radionuclide therapy using ^{177}Lu- and ^{90}Y-labeled somatostatin analogs. J Nucl Med 2005; 46: 13-7.
[PMID: 15653647]

[83]   Häfeli U, Tiefenauer LX, Schbiger PA, Weder HG. A lipophilic complex with ^{186}Re/^{188}Re incorporated in liposomes suitable for radiotherapy. Int J Rad Appl Instrum B 1991; 18(5): 449-54.
[http://dx.doi.org/10.1016/0883-2897(91)90104-S] [PMID: 1670497]

[84]   Emfietzoglou D, Kostarelos K, Sgouros G. An analytic dosimetry study for the use of radionuclide-

liposome conjugates in internal radiotherapy. J Nucl Med 2001; 42(3): 499-504.
[PMID: 11337529]

[85]   Chang CH, Stabin MG, Chang YJ, *et al.* Comparative dosimetric evaluation of nanotargeted [188]Re-(DXR)-liposome for internal radiotherapy. Cancer Biother Radiopharm 2008; 23(6): 749-58.
[http://dx.doi.org/10.1089/cbr.2008.0489] [PMID: 19111045]

[86]   Häfeli UO. Magnetically modulated therapeutic systems. Int J Pharm 2004; 277(1-2): 19-24.
[http://dx.doi.org/10.1016/j.ijpharm.2003.03.002] [PMID: 15158965]

[87]   Liang S, Wang Y, Yu J, Zhang C, Xia J, Yin D. Surface modified superparamagnetic iron oxide nanoparticles: as a new carrier for bio-magnetically targeted therapy. J Mater Sci Mater Med 2007; 18(12): 2297-302.
[http://dx.doi.org/10.1007/s10856-007-3130-6] [PMID: 17562137]

[88]   Ruggiero A, Villa CH, Holland JP, *et al.* Imaging and treating tumor vasculature with targeted radiolabeled carbon nanotubes. Int J Nanomed 2010; 5: 783-802.
[http://dx.doi.org/10.2147/IJN.S13300] [PMID: 21042424]

[89]   Sun X, Huang X, Yan X, *et al.* Chelator-free ^{64}Cu-integrated gold nanomaterials for positron emission tomography imaging guided photothermal cancer therapy. ACS Nano 2014; 8(8): 8438-46.
[http://dx.doi.org/10.1021/nn502950t] [PMID: 25019252]

[90]   Wang Z, Huang P, Jacobson O, *et al.* Biomineralization-inspired synthesis of copper sulfide-ferritin nanocages as cancer theranostics. ACS Nano 2016; 10(3): 3453-60.
[http://dx.doi.org/10.1021/acsnano.5b07521] [PMID: 26871955]

[91]   Feng Q, Zhang Y, Zhang W, *et al.* Programmed near-infrared light-responsive drug delivery system for combined magnetic tumor-targeting magnetic resonance imaging and chemo-phototherapy. Acta Biomater 2017; 49: 402-13.
[http://dx.doi.org/10.1016/j.actbio.2016.11.035] [PMID: 27890732]

[92]   Zhou M, Chen Y, Adachi M, *et al.* Single agent nanoparticle for radiotherapy and radio-photothermal therapy in anaplastic thyroid cancer. Biomaterials 2015; 57: 41-9.
[http://dx.doi.org/10.1016/j.biomaterials.2015.04.013] [PMID: 25913249]

[93]   Kurihara A, Deguchi Y, Pardridge WM. Epidermal growth factor radiopharmaceuticals: [111]In chelation, conjugation to a blood-brain barrier delivery vector *via* a biotin-polyethylene linker, pharmacokinetics, and *in vivo* imaging of experimental brain tumors. Bioconjug Chem 1999; 10(3): 502-11.
[http://dx.doi.org/10.1021/bc980123x] [PMID: 10346884]

SUBJECT INDEX

www.ingramcontent.com/pod-product-compliance
Lightning Source LLC
Chambersburg PA
CBHW041701210326
41598CB00007B/492